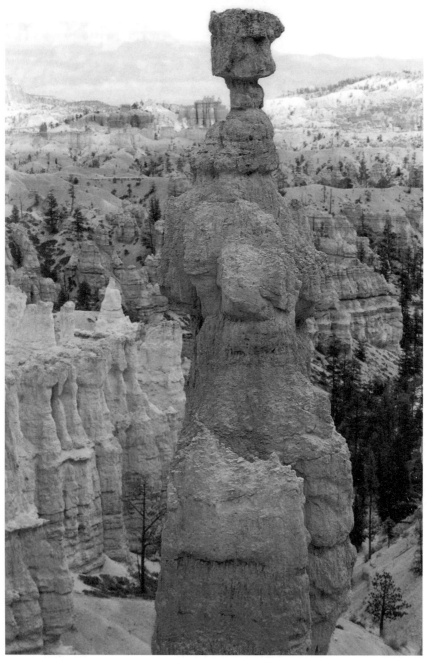

50
BEST
SHORT HIKES
in
Utah's
National
Parks

Ron Adkison

WILDERNESS PRESS
BERKELEY

FIRST EDITION August 2001
Second printing April 2003

Inside photos by Ron Adkison except where noted
Maps by Anthony McDemas at Design Maps
Book design by Kathy Morey
Cover design by Larry B. Van Dyke

Library of Congress Card Number 2001045321
ISBN 0-89997-260-8

Manufactured in the United States of America

Published by **Wilderness Press**
             1200 Fifth Street
             Berkeley, CA 94710
             (800) 443-7227; FAX (510) 558-1696
             mail@wildernesspress.com
             www.wildernesspress.com
Contact us for a free catalog

Front cover photo: *The Zion Narrows, Zion National Park, Utah,*
                   © 2001 Tom Till
Back cover photos: *(top) Hickman Bridge, Capitol Reef National Park,*
                   © 2001 Ron Adkison
                   (bottom) Chesler Park, Canyonlands National Park,
                   © 2001 Ron Adkison
Frontispiece: *Thor's Hammer on Navajo Loop Trail, Bryce National Park,*
              © 2001 Ben Adkison

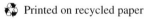 Printed on recycled paper

Library of Congress Cataloging-in-Publication Data
Adkison, Ron.
    50 best short hikes in Utah's national parks : Zion, Bryce, Capitol Reef, Arches,
    Canyonlands / Ron Adkison— 1st ed.
        p. cm.
    Includes bibliographical references and index.
    ISBN 0-89997-260-8
        1. Hiking—Utah—Guidebooks. 2. National parks and reserves—Utah—Guidebooks.
    3. Utah—Guidebooks. I. Title: Fifty best short hikes in Utah's national parks. II. Title.
    GV199.42.U8 A35 2001
    917.9204'34—dc2l
                                                            2001045321

Disclaimer

Hiking in the backcountry entails unavoidable risk that every hiker assumes and must be aware of and respect. The fact that a trail is described in this book is not a representation that it will be safe for you. Trails vary greatly in difficulty and in the degree of conditioning and agility one needs to enjoy them safely. On some hikes, routes may have changed or conditions may have deteriorated since the descriptions were written. Also trail conditions can change from day to day, owing to weather and other factors. A trail that is safe on a dry day or for a highly conditioned, agile, properly equipped hiker may be completely unsafe for someone else or unsafe under adverse weather conditions.

You can minimize your risks on the trail by being knowledgeable, prepared and alert. There is not space in this book for a general treatise on safety in the mountains, but there are a number of good books and public courses on the subject and you should take advantage of them to increase your knowledge. Just as important, you should always be aware of your own limitations and of conditions existing when and where you are hiking. If conditions are dangerous, or if you're not prepared to deal with them safely, choose a different hike! It's better to have wasted a drive than to be the subject of a mountain rescue.

These warnings are not intended to scare you off the trails. Millions of people have safe and enjoyable hikes every year. However, one element of the beauty, freedom and excitement of the wilderness is the presence of risks that do not confront us at home. When you hike you assume those risks. They can be met safely, but only if you exercise your own independent judgement and common sense.

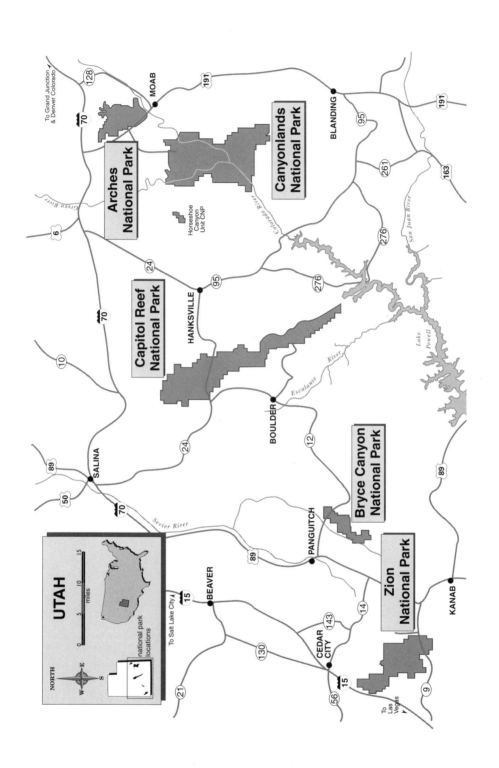

The Hikes

Capitol Reef National Park 81

The Hikes

Arches National Park. 125

The Hikes

Canyonlands National Park 163

The Hikes

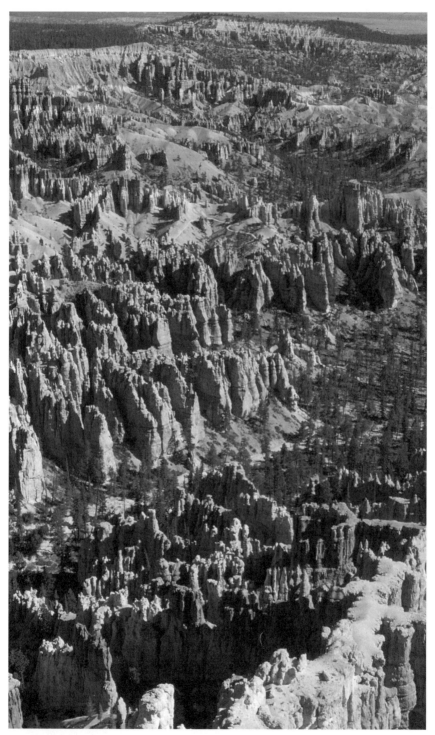

The Bryce Canyon amphitheater from the Peekaboo Loop Trail

Introduction

Five of perhaps the most magnificent national parks in the nation stretch across the southern third of Utah. These parks embrace some of the finest and most unusual examples of erosional forms on the globe, and they are truly among the wonders of the world. Utah's national parks are a veritable wilderness of stone, and indeed much of the land in each park has been recommended for federal wilderness designation. Many serious hikers, however, shun national parks, believing that such areas are tourist meccas where a wilderness experience is difficult, if not impossible, to have. That may be true for some of our national parks, but not for Utah's. Even in Zion National Park, where annual visitation averages more than two million people (nearly half the total annual visitation to all Utah national parks), the hiker can enjoy magnificent, wild country and a good deal of solitude only a short distance from most any road.

The majority of park visitors spend only a day in each Utah park, viewing the scenery from the comfort of their vehicles as they try to see as much country as a one-to-two-week vacation will allow. This book was written to satisfy the needs of short-term visitors—to help them make the most of their park visit, and to choose the short hike that is best for them. Are there really "50 Best" hikes in Utah's National Parks? In the author's opinion, nearly every hike in these parks is "the best." The choice of "50 Best" is based on the author's years of hiking here, and these hikes, ranging from a short stroll of 0.3 mile to an all-day outing of 10.4 miles, sample some of the finest and most diverse landscapes in each park. All hikes are easily accessible, beginning along primary park roads, and they are all well marked and easy to follow. For visitors with limited time, these parks have a great deal to offer. Much of the parks' scenery can be enjoyed from park roadways; numerous short trails, many of them nature trails, offer visitors a chance to stretch their legs, smell the desert's fragrance, feel the wind in their faces, view seemingly endless panoramas and incomparable landscapes, enjoy the delicate blossoms and the perfumes of myriad wildflowers, and observe desert creatures going about their day-to-day lives. Many short trails require no special hiking ability, and some are accessible to handicapped persons in wheelchairs and even to parents pushing baby strollers.

For an extended stay, each park has one or more excellent campgrounds, and some are available to large recreational vehicles. Each park also boasts a visitor center and interpretive activities that include ranger-led hikes and evening-campfire naturalist programs.

Visitors to the majestic landscape of Utah's national parks will enjoy a wide range of scenery, including vast plateaus clothed in cool forests of pine, fir, and aspen; magnificent canyons up to 4000 feet deep; soaring cliffs, some of them sheer and smooth from top to bottom, others broken and fluted with great buttresses and columns; cliff-edged mesas, some capped by stone, others topped by velvety grasslands and "pygmy" forests of pinyon and juniper; broad desert valleys and sun-baked desert flats; domes, crags, arches and pinnacles of solid stone, colored in nearly every shade of the spectrum.

Diverse species of plants and animals compose another aspect of the scenery in Utah's national parks. They live in delicate balance and are adapted to the rigors of the high desert, where rainfall is scant and undependable, and where temperatures can be excessively hot. This desert country of the Colorado Plateau may seem harsh and unforgiving, inhospitable to human life if not to plants and animals; but humans too have lived and even thrived here for thousands of years. Park visitors will encounter granaries and cliff dwellings of the Ancestral Puebloans (formerly called the "Anasazi"), rock-writing panels dating back more than 2000 years, old homesteads, cowboy line camps, and even farm equipment.

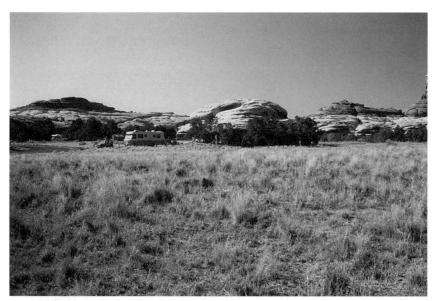

Squaw Flat Campground, Canyonlands National Park

Yes, Utah's national parks have a great deal to offer to everyone, from chapters of natural history and human history to chapters of earth history spanning more than 300 million years. The parks also offer diverse recreational opportunities, from dayhikes to extended backcountry treks, horseback rides (in Zion and Bryce), 4-wheel-drive trips, and river float trips.

How to use the hike descriptions

Here is a brief explanation of the hike description format. A round-trip hike is one on which you retrace your outbound steps. A loop trip involves no retracing. A semiloop trip retraces part of a route after making a loop somewhere along the course.

Elevation gain tells you how much total elevation you will gain on a particular hike, from the time you leave the trailhead to the time you return. Some hikes may be uphill or downhill all the way to the destination, and others may have many ups and downs along the way.

Average hiking time gives a conservative estimate of the time most hikers will spend actually walking on a trail.

The *Difficulty rating* of a given hike is the author's opinion, calculated by taking into account a variety of factors including length of the hike, elevation change, nature of the trail, and availability of shade—all in relation to the average hiker's ability. Difficulty ratings range from 1—a short and very easy walk, to 5—an all-day hike that's guaranteed to provide you with a complete workout.

For parents hiking with children, the *Child rating*, on a scale of 1 to 3, will help you decide which trail is best suited for your family. A trail with a rating of 1 is suitable for your toddler—with supervision; trails with a rating of 2 should be suitable for youngsters in the 6- to 8-year range; and a rating of 3 indicates a trail is too long and/or hazardous for young children, and is more appropriate for well-conditioned kids above the age of 9 or 10.

Best season is the average optimum season in which to hike the trail, including those months with the greatest probability of fair weather and moderate temperatures. Seasons vary from year to year. In some years spring can be quite moist and cool, and in other years spring can be unusually hot and dry; likewise with the months of autumn. Visitors can enjoy the parks year-round, however, they are encouraged to check with the appropriate national-park office prior to their visit to determine likely weather patterns.

Hazards indicate things hikers should be aware of before venturing onto the trail. Only the most pertinent hazards are listed; all hikers are advised to be prepared for a variety of unexpected situations. Lack of water is not mentioned as a hazard, but hikers who take any of the hikes in this book without bringing adequate water can put themselves in danger. Only one hike in this book, Hike 11, the Peekaboo Loop Trail in Bryce Canyon National

Park, has drinking fountains at one point along the trail. Drinking from open water sources without first filtering or otherwise disinfecting the water can lead to serious intestinal disease. Always carry at least 2 quarts of water per person on any of the short hikes in this book. For more information on dehydration and heat-related illness, see the section "Hiking Utah's desert parks," below.

Elevation figures in parentheses within each hike description give the elevation at a particular point. The difference between two consecutive elevations does not necessarily indicate the amount of elevation gain or loss between the two points, as many trails have ups and downs between points.

Geology of the Colorado Plateau

Geologists have subdivided the United States into physiographic provinces, each with its own distinct landscape characteristics, mode of formation, and geologic and geographic patterns. The Colorado Plateau physiographic province is one of the most unusual regions on the globe. This 130,000-square-mile region is a vast highland that lies above lower-elevation regions to the south and west, and abuts the higher country of the central and southern Rocky Mountains to the north and east.

Flat-lying rock beds, mostly of sedimentary origin, characterize the plateau. However, geological periods of folding, uplift, and erosion created an irregular surface. Great blocks of the plateau have been uplifted along faults, forming the High Plateaus upon which Bryce Canyon and Zion are situated. Folds, anticlines, and synclines in the earth's crust are largely responsible for the incomparable scenery in Capitol Reef, Arches, and Canyonlands national parks. Two erosional forms typify the Colorado Plateau. Mesas (meaning tables in Spanish) are remnant segments of the plateau isolated by erosion, which are generally flat on top and bounded by steep cliffs. Buttes are smaller, cliff-edged prominences, with or without a flat top, that have been completely isolated and are detached from the main body of a mesa.

Sedimentary rocks are dominant in the national parks of Utah and the Colorado Plateau as a whole, with only a few scattered outcrops of igneous and metamorphic rocks. Most of the sedimentary strata in the region are flat-lying and in the same sequence in which they were laid down. Since the climate of the region is dry, little soil and vegetational cover have developed. Moreover, downcutting of the canyons has exposed the full sequence of sedimentary rocks deposited on the Colorado Plateau. Geologists can read this rock record and learn much about the climate and the environmental conditions that prevailed when the sediments were laid down. The presence of fossils here also increases our understanding of the development of life on the ever-changing earth.

More than 300 million years have elapsed since the rocks exposed in Utah's national parks were deposited. The region included, at various times in the past, sea floors, floodplains, river deltas, swamps, coastal marshes and lagoons, sea coasts, and vast arid deserts. Yet nowhere in the geologic record is there an indication that the region earlier contained the great canyon systems it does today. Around the periphery of the plateau great mountains were uplifted and then eroded away, and other areas of the land in the plateau's interior subsided into basins and low-lying areas that were periodically inundated by seas or freshwater lake systems.

Following regional uplift of the Colorado Plateau about 10–15 million years ago, erosion by the Colorado River and its tributaries stripped away much of the thousands of feet of lithified (made into rock) sediments, exhuming older strata that had been buried by younger sediments for millions of years. Today, weathering—whereby rocks are broken down into their constituent materials—and erosion—whereby these materials are carried away by wind and running water—are the principal earth-shaping processes affecting the land in the Colorado Plateau.

Formation of arches

Two categories of arches adorn Utah's national parks: those with an opening below or behind the arch, and those without openings. Arches without openings, such as the many large arches that are found high on massive sandstone walls in Zion National Park, are not considered in this discussion. Neither are natural bridges, because they are not common in Utah's national parks. Natural bridges, unlike arches, are formed by a meandering stream that cuts laterally into a narrow fin of rock, eventually cutting a hole through it. Aptly named Natural Bridges National Monument, in southeast Utah, is the best place to see those phenomena.

Arches with openings are relatively rare in the world, but are common on the Colorado Plateau, and all of Utah's national parks display stunning examples. There are two very common types of arches with openings in Utah's parks: 1) arches in a thin, vertical wall—or fin—of sandstone; they have a vertical opening entirely below the span; and 2) pothole arches, which have a horizontal opening. Chemical and physical weathering processes create both types of arches.

In the first type, the process of arch formation begins when groundwater seeps down through a porous sandstone layer and encounters an impermeable layer, such as shale. The groundwater then seeps outward along this interface of layers, and eventually reaches the face of a cliff. There it dissolves the natural cement that binds sand grains into stone, and then water, wind, and gravity remove the sand grains. Thus a small indentation begins to form on the cliff face at the horizontal interface of the two layers. This indentation grows horizontally and vertically as the rock immediately above the indentation is undercut and destabilized, and eventually breaks away.

Over time, more rockfall on a small or grand scale causes the arch to grow. The indentation becomes larger, forming what is called an alcove. If the body of rock behind the cliff is narrow enough, like the fins in Arches and Canyonlands national parks, the alcove will continue to penetrate the rock until it reaches the other side, and an opening forms. If two alcoves form on opposite sides of the fin, an opening develops much more rapidly.

The second type of arch, a pothole arch, is the most common type in Capitol Reef and Canyonlands national parks. A pothole arch begins to form when water collects in a pothole on top of a sandstone cliff and close to the cliff face. Although much of the water trapped in a pothole evaporates, some seeps down into the porous sandstone below. When this groundwater reaches an impermeable layer, it seeps outward along the interface to the cliff face, and an alcove eventually forms there, in the same way as described above. The alcove and the pothole continue to enlarge, and they eventually coalesce, forming a nearly horizontal opening called a pothole arch.

Utah's national parks are as diverse as they are beautiful. But what they all have in common are their colorful, magnificently sculpted rocks, which make these parks some of the finest scenic attractions in the world. The effects of erosion on more than two dozen different sedimentary rock formations have made the landscapes of the parks exciting and dramatic.

To learn more about the geology of Utah's national parks, choose from a wide variety of publications at each park visitor center.

Desert flora

The national parks of Utah are home to hundreds of species of plants, despite an arid to semiarid climate, high temperatures in summer and bitter cold in winter, a lack of dependable precipitation, and poorly developed soil cover. Each plant occupies its own niche in the desert, growing only in a habitat that meets its specific environmental requirements.

It is beyond the scope of this guide to catalog all or even many of the hundreds of plant species visitors are likely to encounter in Utah's national parks, but the trail descriptions do identify certain plants at various locations. Anyone interested in learning more about desert flora can obtain one or more of the excellent books on the subject at any park visitor center.

Desert plants have developed various methods to cope with the desert's extreme climate. Some plants, those that grow in riparian woodlands and hanging gardens (assemblages of water-loving plants found on canyon walls), are hardy enough to withstand the desert's extreme heat, but can survive only where a continuous supply of surface or underground moisture is available. These plants could be called drought-escaping.

Phreatophytes are plants that have evolved deep, extensive root systems to survive the extreme lack of moisture that characterizes most desert environments. This root system enables them to tap underground sources of moisture. Once their roots reach the water table, their growth is not dependent on rainfall.

Most desert plants are xerophytes. Xerophytes include succulent plants, which have fleshy leaves or stems that store water for extended periods. Cacti are an example of a succulent xerophyte; they have shallow and often widespread root systems that absorb soil moisture from even the lightest rainfall. Cacti are leafless, and their succulent pads are actually stems. These stems swell with stored moisture in spring, and they slowly and economically metabolize that moisture throughout the dry part of the year. When most of the moisture has been used, the pads shrink and become wrinkled; unlike nonsucculent xerophytes, cacti do not go dormant when stressed by drought.

Nonsucculent xerophytes have evolved a number of characteristics, other than water storage, which help them survive long periods of drought. Deep root systems and special cellular structures help them suck moisture from the soil long after rain has fallen. The leaves of many xerophytes are vertically oriented, reducing the surface area exposed directly to sunlight and thus retarding water-loss and excessive heating. Some leaves have a waxy or resinous coating that slows moisture evaporation. Densely matted hairs and a grayish pigment function in reducing evaporation and reflecting sunlight. Small pores on some leaves also decreases the amount of water that escapes from the plant.

Plants in desert climates are often widely spaced, limiting competition for the little available water. Some plants conserve energy and moisture by curling their leaves or even dropping them. If there is not enough moisture to support the plant, then all but perhaps a single branch will die back; or the entire above-ground part of the plant may die, all of its energies diverted to preserve the life-sustaining root system.

Many xerophytes have also developed characteristics to protect themselves from predators. Rigid, woody, and/or spiny branches discourage browsing animals from eating them, especially when combined with hairy or resinous foliage.

In most mountainous regions in the western U.S., plants are fairly evenly separated into belts, or zones, that vary with elevation, temperature and precipitation. However, the plant communities of the Colorado Plateau are not uniform in their patterns; the land itself is likewise highly varied, containing deep and sometimes moist canyons, parched mesas and desert flats, vast expanses of naked stone, and sheer cliffs devoid of vegetation and soil.

For example, the pinyon-juniper woodland is one of the most common plant communities visitors will encounter, but this woodland does not grow at any typical elevation; rather, it grows where local environmental conditions are suitable to support it. In Zion National Park, for example, one will find this woodland growing at 4000 feet, while near Canyonlands it is found above 7000. Where a canyon has been eroded into the plateau, one may also find a pinyon-juniper woodland, while on the plateau above the canyon only a scattering of shrubs may exist.

Hiking Utah's desert parks

The unique landscapes of rock and sand, canyons and mesas that make up the high desert of the Colorado Plateau offer some of the finest, most remote and most awe-inspiring wilderness hiking in the nation. But to enjoy this magical country to the fullest, and to minimize your impact on the land—and the land's potential impact on you—pretrip planning and an awareness of the special hazards involved in a desert trek are imperative, even for short dayhikes.

Utah's high-desert national parks are arid to semiarid, meaning that an average of 15 inches of moisture or less falls annually. Often an entire month's share of precipitation falls in a few hours or a single day. Humidity is very low, and summer heat is intense. Daily temperature fluctuations of 30 to 50° between daytime highs and nighttime lows are not uncommon. Surface water is scarce, and much of it is highly mineralized and not potable. Many trails are rugged, and some require the use of hands to scramble over steep slickrock—bare, smooth sandstone.

The trails in Utah's national parks sample virtually every aspect of the park landscapes, from wooded mesas and forested plateaus to open desert flats, cliffs, and deep, cavernous defiles. Many trails follow canyon bottoms, where the hiker may encounter deep sand or be forced to wade through waist-deep waters or even swim across deep pools. Some trails are accessible only to the adventurous wilderness enthusiast with basic rock-climbing ability, while others can be trod by visitors who have never before set foot on a trail. Still other "trails" are mere routes over slickrock, marked only by cairns—small piles of rocks.

Hiking over slickrock can be a joy, but it is not without its hazards. Loosened sand grains can make slickrock somewhat slippery, but even steep slickrock usually provides good traction, except when wet. However, when snow-covered, smooth sandstone is extremely treacherous and should be avoided.

A trip into Utah's deserts is not a life-threatening survival situation, but one must be prepared to meet challenges and to confront emergency situations if they arise. In most areas of the national parks in Utah, help is usually not far away. But in more remote areas, such as the Waterpocket District in Capitol Reef or the Kolob Terrace in Zion, emergency assistance is distant. Proper planning and recognition of hazards and of one's abilities are your best insurance for a safe and enjoyable outing.

Plan your trip in advance, including possible sidetrips. Leave your itinerary with a friend or relative, and have them notify the appropriate park office if you don't return when expected. It is easy to get sidetracked into exploring hidden canyons and mesas in the Utah desert, but try to stick to your planned route.

Hiking alone in the desert is unwise, but many people do it. If you hike alone, you must take great care not to become lost, and to avoid situations which might result in injury. When hiking with a group, set the pace according to the slowest member, and stay together. Don't exceed the limits of your capabilities or those of others in your group. Before climbing steep rock, ask yourself if you are making a wise decision. Don't climb up anything that you may not be able to get back down, and vice versa.

Above all, hikers should try to minimize their impact on the fragile desert landscape.

Equipment for desert hiking

Many hikers are unsure of what type of footwear to use in the desert. Some hikers wear jogging shoes, but these offer no ankle support or protection from thorny plants. Rigid lug-sole boots don't provide adequate traction on slickrock. Instead, consider wearing lightweight, breathable hiking boots. These offer ankle support and have a softer, more flexible sole for better traction. For hikes that require much wading or frequent stream crossings where your feet will be constantly wet (such as in Zion Narrows if you hike beyond the end of Riverside Walk), running shoes or sandals may seem like the best choice for footwear, but they are not. To provide adequate support and protection for your feet while hiking in wet conditions, consider wearing an older pair of boots, a pair you are willing to sacrifice to get you safely and comfortably through your trip.

Even in the desert, it is advisable to carry raingear, as storms can happen at any time, and often develop unexpectedly. Several carnivorous insects, including sand flies, mosquitoes, and especially the tiny, black, gnatlike flies called midges (no-see-ums), constantly harass hikers from early spring through midsummer. Strong insect repellents, preferably some natural product, are effective against mosquitoes, and to a lesser extent against flesh-eating sand flies, but these products seem to have little effect on midges. The only product that deters midges for most people is a bath-oil spray from Avon called Skin-so-Soft.

Hiking seasons

One can hike in Utah's national parks throughout the year, except in Bryce Canyon, where winter snowpack renders that park accessible only to cross-country skiers or snowshoers. Many visitors take their vacations during summer, but since summers in the Utah desert are very hot, it is not the most desirable time to visit here. The high country of Bryce Canyon and parts of Zion, where summers are pleasantly warm, are the exceptions. Hot summer conditions usually invade the Utah desert by mid-June, although in some years summer may begin earlier. Daily high temperatures of 90 to 100° are common, with occasional spells of 110° heat. Nighttime lows typically dip to the 60s or 70s, but areas with abundant slickrock continue to radiate heat long into the night. Usually by late July the thunderstorm, or monsoon, season begins, bringing the threat of heavy downpours, high winds, lightning, and flash floods. Some summers, however, are quite dry, while others are uncommonly wet, but thunderstorms usually begin to abate by mid-September.

Autumn typically boasts some of the clearest, most stable weather of the year, and is perhaps the most delightful season to visit the Utah desert. Daily maximum temperatures range from the 70s and 80s in September to the 40s and 50s in late November and December. Overnight lows are typically in the 20- to 50°- range. Storms are possible, but are usually of short duration. However, snow may begin to fall in October, and becomes increasingly likely by late November and December, as temperatures drop and Pacific storms become more vigorous.

Although the chances of snowfall increase during winter, snow cover is generally light and rarely lasts more than a few days except in sheltered recesses. January and February are often the driest months of the year, with daytime highs ranging from the 20s to the 40s, and overnight lows ranging in the teens and 20s, rarely dipping below zero. But above 7000 feet, and particularly in the high country of Zion and Bryce, temperatures are much colder and snowpack is often heavy.

Spring weather is typically more unstable than winter, with wide variations in temperature and precipitation. March usually brings an onset of spring weather, but occasional Pacific storms produce winds, clouds, rain, and possibly snow as late as April. Most often, spring storms are characterized by showers, sometimes with sunny periods in between. The weather is generally delightful during spring, with daytime highs averaging from the 50s to the 70s, and nighttime lows ranging from 30 to 50°.

In general, visitation to Utah's national parks increases during spring, often reaching a peak around Memorial Day, slackening slightly during summer, and then increasing again around Labor Day.

Heat and safety

Hiking in the Utah desert is especially challenging during the summer, and hikers must take special precautions to avoid heat and water-related injuries. However, adequate water *and* electrolyte consumption is crucial at all times of the year for a safe and enjoyable backcountry excursion.

Park literature tells visitors they must drink one gallon of water per day, regardless of the season. But experienced desert rats know that summer hiking increases that requirement, and they drink at least six quarts of water per day to avoid dehydration. Remember the maxim, "Ration sweat, not water" when hiking in the desert and drink often, not just when you feel thirsty, and particularly during meals and during the cooler hours. During hot weather, rest 10 minutes every hour, and hike only in the morning hours before noon and in the late afternoon, after about 5 or 6 o'clock. During midday, find a shady niche, perhaps in an alcove or beneath an overhanging ledge, and rest until the heat begins to abate and the shadows fall.

When you exercise during the heat of a summer day, you increase the chance that your body may not effectively be able to maintain cooling and circulation. Heat cramps, heat exhaustion, and in the worst case heat stroke may result. Your body expends an enormous amount of energy keeping you cool while hiking in hot weather. You will sweat about one-half to one quart or more of water and electrolytes every hour while hiking in the heat; but since desert air is so dry, sweat may evaporate almost instantly, making its loss nearly imperceptible. Do not wait until you feel thirsty to start replacing lost fluid and electrolytes; by the time you feel thirsty you are already dehydrated.

Your body can absorb only about one quart of fluid per hour, so drink one-half to one quart of water mixed with an electrolyte replacement (Gatorade or Gookinaid) every hour while hiking in the heat. Drinking too much liquid and not replacing electrolytes, however, can lead to a dangerous medical condition known as hyponatremia, or water intoxication, which, if left untreated, can result in seizures and possibly death. To help replace electrolytes, and to supply your body with adequate energy to keep you cool, it is critical that you eat well. During a long hike through desert heat you must eat a lot more food than you normally do (at least double your normal intake of calories), since you will be expending enormous amounts of energy. While hiking, eat small amounts of foods containing complex carbohydrates (breads, fruits, crackers, grains, no-fat energy bars, etc.). Avoid foods high in fats and proteins since these take longer to digest and may unsettle your stomach in the heat.

A moderate level of dehydration (fluid and electrolyte loss) can lead to heat cramps and heat exhaustion. Heat cramps usually develop in the arms and legs after exertion, causing painful muscle spasms. Heat exhaustion, which occurs as the body diverts blood away from internal organs to the skin to cool it, is more serious. Symptoms include cool and clammy skin, perhaps nausea and weakness, and rapid, shallow breathing. If you heed the warning signs, heat exhaustion need not be dangerous. As with heat cramps, immediately cease activity, rest or lie in the shade, loosen clothing, and drink water. If you must resume activity, you should begin slowly.

Heat stroke can result from a moderate-to-large loss of fluid and electrolytes, and is a serious medical emergency that can be fatal if not recognized and treated immediately. Heat stroke involves the temporary shutdown of sweat glands, so the body is unable to cool itself through evaporation. Though heat stroke is uncommon, you should learn to recognize the symptoms. These initially include hot, dry, flushed skin, dry mouth, headache, dizziness and nausea, followed by rapid, shallow breathing, muscular twitching, convulsions, and unconsciousness.

If you suspect heat stroke, you must rapidly cool the victim and immediately seek medical attention. Remove the victim's clothing, and cool by immersion in water or by covering with wet cloths, while fanning continuously to help dissipate body heat. Massage the extremities gently to help increase blood flow and heat loss. Continue these methods until medical assistance arrives or, if unavailable, until the victim begins to recover. The victim should rest under care until he or she is feeling better, and should resume physical activity slowly.

Sunburn is possible at any time of the year, and hikers should take the appropriate precautions. Wear loose-fitting, light-colored clothing that will reflect the heat. Though long pants and long-sleeved shirts are preferable and help reduce dehydration, many hikers wear shorts. Sunscreen is then a must. Wear a hat that will shade the eyes and ears, and use sunglasses to avoid the intense glare reflecting from slickrock. Avoid licking your lips if they are dry, as this will cause splitting, and instead apply lip balm.

Flash floods

Many hiking routes are restricted to canyon bottoms, so keep in mind the possibility of flash floods. Whenever hiking in a canyon, keep an eye out for escape routes to higher ground. Many canyons in the national parks gather their waters beyond park boundaries, so even during sunny weather in your location, a vigorous, isolated thunderstorm miles away could send a roiling wall of water down your canyon. If you hear an increasing roar up-canyon, signaling oncoming floodwaters, seek higher ground immediately, and do not attempt to outrun rushing waters: it cannot be done.

Water safety

In all Utah national parks, rangers and park literature recommend treatment of backcountry water sources. Since this book is for dayhikers, it is strongly recommended that hikers carry all the water they will need, rather than obtaining water from backcountry sources that must be purified before drinking. Most hikes in this book are short, and in cool weather hikers may need to carry only one quart of water. On the longer hikes, at least two, and preferably three quarts should be carried by each hiker. In hot weather, hikers will need to carry even more water to help ensure a safe and enjoyable trip.

Desert creatures

The Utah desert does have its share of biting and sometimes poisonous creatures. The aforementioned sand flies, or deer flies, are common in sandy washes, but mosquitoes are much less common, usually found only near water. Midges, however, are ubiquitous in all the national parks, and they inflict an itching bite even more irritating than the mosquito's. Tarantulas, though large and dangerous-looking, rarely bite unless provoked, but their strong jaws can inflict a painful bite. Their poison is mild, but a bacterial infection can result. The giant desert hairy scorpion is also threatening in its appearance, but its sting is harmless except for being painful. Black widow spiders are common but rarely seen due to their secretive nature. Take care when lifting rocks, as these creatures may be lurking underneath, and always empty your boots or shoes each morning, as spiders and scorpions are attracted to their warmth and moisture.

Finally, poisonous snakes are feared more than any other creature in the desert. The small midget faded rattlesnake occurs in Capitol Reef, Arches, and Canyonlands, where the Hopi rattlesnake also dwells. In Bryce Canyon is the five-foot Great Basin rattlesnake, and in Zion, the western rattlesnake. Overall, sightings of rattlesnakes are rare; hikers are more likely to encounter a rattler in Bryce Canyon than in any other Utah park. When a hiker approaches, a rattlesnake will either slither away and hide, or coil in defense. Many rattle a warning, but some do not. Pay attention to where you place your hands and feet, especially when hiking in brushy or rocky areas. Don't panic if you are bitten; remain calm and still. Exercise only serves to transport the venom more rapidly through your body. People rarely succumb to the bite of a rattlesnake, even without the benefit of any first-aid treatment. The traditional cut-and-suck method has been found to have little value, and can actually increase your chances of infection. A rattlesnake bite results in immediate pain accompanied by swelling. If you are the victim, one of your companions should tie a constricting band above the bite and the swelling, and remove it for 1 minute during every 15-minute period.

Remain calm and quiet, and drink plenty of water. A companion should immediately go to the nearest trailhead or ranger station for help. If you are alone, you should proceed slowly to the nearest location where people are likely to be.

Reducing your impact on the desert

While the desert appears to be a durable landscape, it is actually delicate and fragile, and plant and animal life can be easily disrupted, even by walking off of established trails for only a short distance. Throughout your travels in the Utah desert, you will surely notice a black, crusty covering on bare ground, primarily on clay soils. This ground cover is an assemblage of lower plants, called a microbiotic or a cryptobiotic crust. The crust, made up of mosses, lichens, cyanobacteria (blue-green algae), and fungus in various combinations, is easily destroyed by feet and by vehicle tires, and it may take 25 years to recover. When you walk on this black, lumpy crust, you are destroying plants and hastening wind and water erosion. To reduce your impact on this fragile association of crusty plants, stay on the trails or, if you're hiking cross-country, hike in washes or on slickrock as much as possible, or on soils free of cryptobiotic crusts. If you must hike off-trail through areas of cryptobiotic crust, walk single-file, each member of the group stepping in the footprints ahead of them.

Another important aspect of the national-park experience in Utah is the historic sites, such as Ancestral Puebloan structures and rock writing. Encountering a cliff dwelling, a granary or a rock-writing panel left behind by a long-vanished culture hundreds or even thousands of years ago is one of the special joys of hiking in the Utah desert, and these reminders of ancient desert dwellers lend an air of mystery to the enchanting landscape. Yet with each passing year, vandals, and even well-intentioned but misguided hikers, destroy parts of these valuable resources and remove artifacts from archaeological sites.

It is our responsibility to protect these sites, not only for their scientific value but for ourselves and those who come after. Structures are fragile and crumble easily; do not climb on them. Skin oils destroy pigments on pictograph panels, so restrain the urge to touch them. Do not add graffiti to rock-writing panels. Avoid picking up potsherds, bones, or other lithic scatter at cultural sites. Well-intentioned hikers often pick up artifacts from the ground and place them on display on so-called "museum rocks" at cultural sites. Leave archaeological sites as you found them, preserving the sense of discovery for those who follow. Even walking around a dwelling or other site may destroy cultural resources.

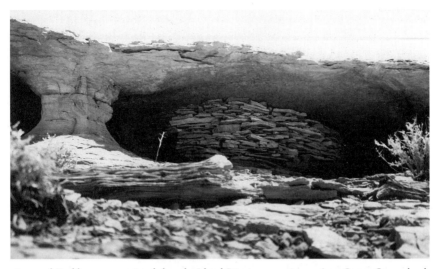

Ancestral Puebloan granary just below the Island District mesa rim on Aztec Butte, Canyonlands National Park

Every artifact—a kernel of corn or a potsherd—provides an important link to the past. Once an artifact is removed or disturbed, it becomes merely an object that cannot be related to its context. The Antiquities Act of 1906 and the Archaeological Resources Protection Act of 1979 make it unlawful to remove, damage, excavate, deface or alter the material remains of human life and activity over 100 years old. There are also state laws protecting cultural resources. Civil and criminal penalties are enforced, and rewards of up to $500 are provided for information leading to the arrest and conviction of offenders.

There are many ways hikers can reduce their impact on the fragile desert. Although techniques of no-trace behavior are now largely common practice among hikers, we occasionally need reminders. In addition to the suggestions above, hikers should keep noise to a minimum, as sound carries far in the desert and echoes among rocks and canyon walls. Keep group size as small as possible—consider splitting your group into smaller parties while hiking. When traveling cross-country, spread out instead of walking single file and concentrating your impact (except when travelling across cryptobiotic crusts).

Always carry out your trash or garbage. In the arid desert climate, things like orange and banana peels will not decompose; rather, they become mummified. Hikers are required to pack out used toilet paper in all of Utah's national parks, even dayhikers. Self-sealing plastic bags are useful for this, and should be standard equipment in every hiker's pack.

Respect plant and animal life in the desert. Moving a stone, uprooting a plant, or killing an undesirable creature disrupts the delicate balance that desert life has achieved. Above all, remember that you are a visitor in the home of plants and animals, so behave as you would in someone's home and act with respect for all desert dwellers.

Driving in Utah's national parks

Most trailheads in the national parks of Utah lie along paved park roads and are accessible to any vehicle, but some lie along remote dirt roads. Dirt roads are often impassable to even 4WD vehicles during and shortly after a heavy rain, when clay beds become a sticky, slippery mess. If you return from a hike to find your dirt road wet from heavy rains, be prepared to wait a day or more for the roadbed to dry. Some roads follow canyons that are subject to dangerous flash floods, which can wash out roads and deposit rocks and other debris on the roadbed. Always check the current road conditions at park visitor centers.

Everyone traveling off main roads should be sure to have a full tank of gas and perhaps some extra, at least 5 gallons of water, a shovel, extra food and clothing, a tow line, and a tire pump. On rough or flood-damaged roads, a little shovel work can save you hours of down-time should your vehicle become stuck or damaged.

Be sure to check road conditions and weather forecasts before driving off main roads, and when in doubt, stop your vehicle and scout ahead on foot; a few minutes of scouting may save you hours of digging out.

Park regulations

The mission of the National Park Service is to preserve the natural and historical values within national parks, while providing for the enjoyment of the landscape in a manner that will leave it unimpaired for future generations. We can all assist by following the guidelines established by park managers. Observing these regulations need not hinder our outdoor experiences, and in fact most of them embody common-sense behavior. Though these regulations are the law of the land in our national parks, we should choose to employ techniques of no trace not only in the parks but wherever we travel.

Below is a general list of regulations that apply to all Utah national parks.

- Backcountry use permits are required for all visitors camping in the backcountry or in 4WD campsites. They are available at all visitor centers, and a fee is required in most of the parks. Rangers will explain pertinent regulations when you obtain your permit.
- Campfires are prohibited except in frontcountry campgrounds.

- Wood gathering is not allowed, so you must bring your own wood for use in campgrounds, and carry a stove in the backcountry.
- Motorized vehicles must be licensed and street-legal, even those used mainly on backcountry 4WD roads. All vehicles, including mountain bikes, are restricted to designated vehicle routes; off-route travel is not permitted. Bicycles are not allowed on any single track trail.
- Visitors are urged to use toilet facilities where available. Otherwise they must bury their waste in a hole 4–6 inches deep, carefully covering it when finished. All of the parks require that backcountry users pack out their toilet paper, and never burn it. Do not bury it, as it will not readily decompose.
- Pets are not permitted in any backcountry roadless area or on hiking trails. They may be transported in vehicles on frontcountry park roads, and may be kept overnight in park campgrounds. Any pet outside of a vehicle must be on a leash less than 6 feet long or otherwise physically constrained at all times. No pet may be left unattended overnight, or left unattended, tied, or physically confined in the frontcountry while you hike.
- All trash and garbage, including used toilet paper, must be packed out of the backcountry. Burial of refuse is not permitted.
- Weapons must be unloaded, broken down and cased during transport in national parks. Weapons of any kind are prohibited in the backcountry. Hunting is also prohibited.
- Observe camping restrictions in regard to water sources and do not use soaps in or near water sources. In most parks, campsites can be established no closer than 300 feet from nonflowing water sources, such as seeps, springs and potholes, and no closer than 100 feet from free-flowing streams. Swimming in potholes is not allowed unless the pothole is continually recharged by flowing water.
- Destruction, defacement, disturbance, or removal of natural or historical objects in national parks is not permitted.

Hiking checklist

The equipment for hiking Utah's desert country is little different from that used in any other wild region. Many of us tend to forget something, especially on backpack trips, but even for a dayhike, be sure you have the following essential items:

What to take in your daypack:
- Water (at least 2 quarts per person for dayhikes)
- First-aid kit (should include bandages, antiseptic, snake-bite kit, constricting band, Ace bandage, anti-inflammatory and/or pain medication, etc.)

- Pocket knife
- Sunglasses (with UV protection)
- Sunscreen (with a SPF of 15 or greater)
- Topographic maps (know or learn how to read them)
- Flashlight (with fresh batteries and spare bulb)
- Extra food and water (even on short hikes)
- Toilet paper (and self-sealing plastic bags to pack out used toilet paper)
- Insect repellent
- Lip balm
- Water bottles (1- to 2-quart Nalgene bottles are best)
- Enough food for your trip (include high energy/high carbohydrate foods)
- Camera, film, lenses, filters
- Binoculars
- Rain parka or poncho
- Rain pants
- Parka, preferably synthetic fleece
- Watch
- Signal mirror
- Rope (for lowering and raising packs over obstacles)

What to wear—depends on temperature:

- Thermal underwear, preferably polypropylene
- Hat, wide-brimmed
- Lightweight, light-colored clothing (use the "layering" method)
- Pants and shorts
- Wool shirt or sweater
- Lightweight hiking boots
- Socks

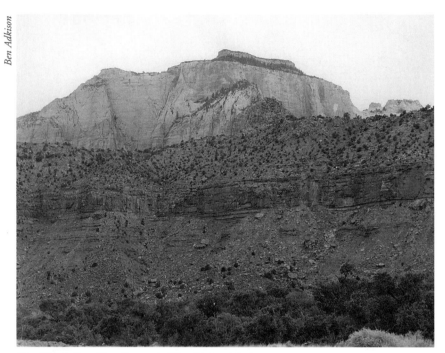

West Temple from Zion Canyon in Zion National Park

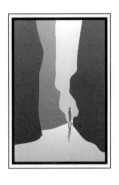

Zion National Park

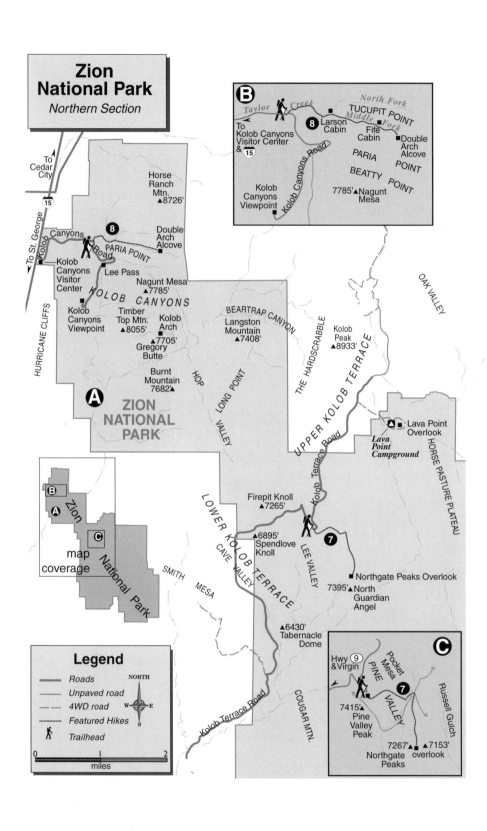

Zion National Park
Northern Section

To Cedar City

15

To St. George

Horse Ranch Mtn. ▲8726'

Kolob Canyons Road

8

PARIA POINT

Double Arch Alcove

Kolob Canyons Visitor Center

Lee Pass

Nagunt Mesa ▲7785'

KOLOB CANYONS

HURRICANE CLIFFS

Kolob Canyons Viewpoint

Timber Top Mtn. ▲8055'

Kolob Arch ▲7705'

Gregory Butte

Burnt Mountain 7682'▲

BEARTRAP CANYON

Langston Mountain ▲7408'

THE HARDSCRABBLE

Kolob Peak ▲8933'

OAK VALLEY

A

ZION NATIONAL PARK

HOP VALLEY

LONG POINT VALLEY

UPPER KOLOB TERRACE

Kolob Terrace Road

Lava Point Overlook

Lava Point Campground

HORSE PASTURE PLATEAU

B
A

C

map coverage

Zion National Park

SMITH MESA

LOWER KOLOB TERRACE

CAVE VALLEY

Firepit Knoll ▲7265'

▲6895' Spendlove Knoll

LEE VALLEY

7

Northgate Peaks Overlook

7395'▲ North Guardian Angel

▲6430' Tabernacle Dome

COUGAR MTN.

Kolob Terrace Road

Legend

—— *Roads*
—— *Unpaved road*
- - - *4WD road*
····· *Featured Hikes*
🚶 *Trailhead*

NORTH
W — E
S

0   1   2
miles

B

Taylor Creek

North Fork

Middle Fork

TUCUPIT POINT

8

Larson Cabin

Fife Cabin

Double Arch Alcove

To Kolob Canyons Visitor Center & 15

Kolob Canyons Road

Kolob Canyons Viewpoint

PARIA POINT

BEATTY POINT

7785'▲Nagunt Mesa

C

Hwy 9 & Virgin

Pocket Mesa

PINE VALLEY

7

7415'▲ Pine Valley Peak

Russell Gulch

7267'▲ Northgate Peaks

▲7153' overlook

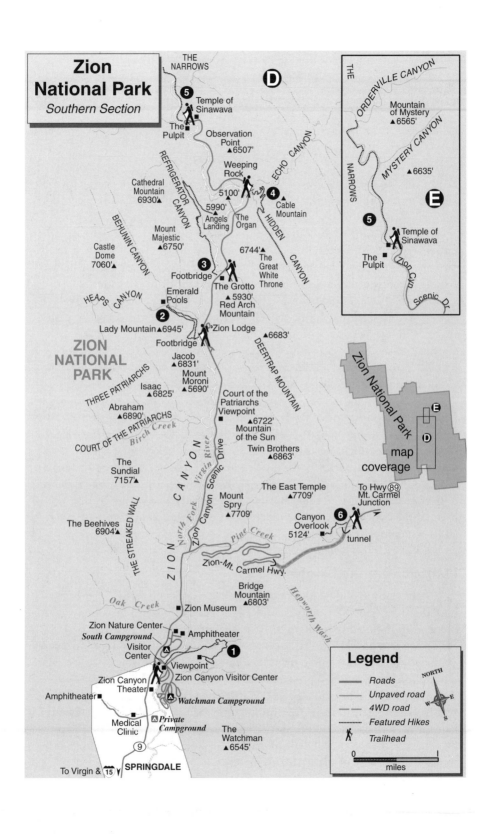

Introduction

In the far southwestern corner of Utah, very near where the Colorado Plateau meets the mountains and valleys of the Great Basin, lies Zion National Park, one of the gems of the national park system.

Zion's 147,000 acres contain landscapes of incredible beauty and infinite diversity. Sculptured cliffs tower thousands of feet above deeply incised canyons and display a kaleidoscope of pastel hues; their color and brilliance change before viewers' eyes with the changing light of the day.

Zion National Park encompasses the Kolob Terrace, the part of the vast Markagunt Plateau that forms the Virgin River watershed, southwest Utah's largest tributary to the Colorado River. The Hurricane Cliffs bound the plateau on the west, forming the boundary between two major physiographic provinces: the Basin and Range Province to the west, and the Colorado Plateau stretching eastward to the Rocky Mountains.

The North Fork of the Virgin has created a deep and narrow canyon of incomparable beauty. At its widest point, one-third mile separates the canyon walls, and at its narrowest, only 20 feet or so. Imposing buttes and towering crags crown the canyon's cliffs, and from below they appear to be majestic mountain peaks. From the heights of the gently contoured plateau, however, viewers gain a different perspective of them. Up there, one quickly notices that the tops of these buttes and towering crags were at one time parts of the continuous level landscape of the plateau. They are now isolated from it simply by erosion.

Plants and animals of Zion

Zion is home to 670 species of flowering plants and ferns, 95 species of mammals, 30 species of reptiles, and 125 species of birds. This vast array of life in Zion helps dispel the myth that a desert is barren and lifeless. True, the region is semiarid, annual precipitation ranging from slightly more than 15 inches in the canyon to an estimated 21 inches atop the plateaus. But despite searing summer heat, Zion has a relative abundance of water—more than any other Utah national park. More than a dozen canyons boast perennial streams, many nurtured by springs that issue from the Navajo Sandstone, a thick and porous layer that is a virtual stone reservoir. Not only do these streams provide delightful haunts for hikers, but their presence promotes the diversity of plant and animal life.

Elevations in the park range from 3666 feet to 8740 feet and represent a wide range of vegetation. A *life zone* is a biogeographical region, defined by the plant communities that typically live within its elevation and precipitation range. Life zones often overlap altitudinally, because particular combinations of soil cover and exposure to sunlight create microclimates here and there. For example, the Transition Life Zone in Zion contains the ponderosa-pine and mountain-brush plant communities, and occasionally members of the fir and aspen communities as well.

The altitudinal range of Zion supports plant communities from sparse desert shrubs to cool forests of pine, fir and aspen. In the Lower Sonoran Zone, blackbrush, yucca, and various species of cacti—mostly prickly-pear and beavertail cactus—dominate the shrublands. The Upper Sonoran Zone occurs mostly in the lower-to-mid-elevations of the park, on drier sites. Single-leaf pinyon and Utah juniper distinguish the pinyon-juniper woodland and are the dominant tree species in this zone, well adapted to heat and drought. Gambel oak often appears in the pinyon-juniper woodland, and it forms oak woodlands in wetter, protected sites in the canyons. Two-needle pinyon and Utah juniper dominate on mid-elevation slopes. Typical shrubs in the Upper Sonoran Zone include buffaloberry, Utah serviceberry, squaw-bush, broom snakeweed, rabbitbrush, and shrub live oak. Littleleaf mountain mahogany, very similar in appearance to blackbrush, grows almost exclusively on slickrock in the upper limits of the zone.

The Transition Zone is dominated by stands of ponderosa pine. Gambel oak intermingles with the pines on plateaus and sometimes forms extensive thickets. Bigtooth maple is common in some areas of this zone, enlivening the landscape with red or orange foliage after the first autumn frosts. On well-drained sites, Rocky Mountain juniper mixes among pine forests. Mountain meadows form in poorly drained sites on the plateaus, and groves of quaking aspen fill even wetter sites. Greenleaf manzanita, alderleaf mountain mahogany, snowberry, and big sagebrush are dominant shrubs here.

The Canadian Zone is limited to well-watered slopes in the park's higher elevations, particularly near Lava Point and the buttes rising above the Kolob Canyons. White fir is the dominant tree here, while Douglas-fir occurs in the coolest, most protected sites. These trees are also found on sheltered sites far below on canyon walls where cooler microclimates prevail. Ponderosa pine is present, but in lesser numbers than in the Transition Zone.

Riparian vegetation grows along streams in most of Zion's life zones. Fremont cottonwood is the dominant riparian tree; velvet ash, boxelder and netleaf hackberry add diversity to these areas, including the North Fork Virgin River, and isolated patches along washes where water lies close to the surface.

Another water-loving plant community is the hanging garden community. These unusual sylvan oases grow on moist cliffs throughout Zion. Due to Zion's abundant seeps and springs, they are more widespread here than in any other Utah national park.

Zion's diversity is as well represented by its animal life as it is by its plant life. Reptiles are by far the most frequently encountered animals on Zion's trails. These cold-blooded creatures are especially well-adapted to living in a semiarid environment. Of the 30 species of reptiles occurring in Zion, hikers will most commonly see the eastern fence lizard, likely doing "pushups" on a trailside boulder. Short-horned lizards and western skinks are also common.

The mule deer is one of the most common large mammals in Zion; they range from Zion Canyon to the plateaus. Other mammals include the seldom-seen mountain lion, the mule deer's chief predator. Occasionally, a Rocky Mountain elk wanders into the park from the higher plateau to the north. Striped and spotted skunks, gray foxes, ringtails, mountain voles, and several species of bats also live in Zion, although they are rarely seen.

A vast array of birds visits Zion, representing 271 species, of which 125 remain year-round. Amphibians, of which only seven species occur in Zion, are infrequently seen, since they stay close to water sources and damp areas.

Snails are an important part of Zion's aquatic community. Most noteworthy is the Zion snail, a tiny invertebrate about the size of a pinhead. Endemic to Zion, this snail lives only along seeps and springs on the canyon walls of the Zion Narrows. Finally, many hikers are well acquainted with the most abundant of life forms in the park, insects. Mosquitoes, no-see-ums, and biting flies are real nuisances in spring and early summer, and in some locations these annoying creatures persist well into autumn.

Interpretive activities

Everyone's first stop in Zion should be at the visitor center. Books, maps, backcountry permits for overnight hiking, weather reports, interpretive displays, and schedules of interpretive programs are available there. Park rangers on duty are veritable encyclopedias of information. Zion's visitor center is the largest and most complete such facility in all of Utah's national parks, and your experience in the park will be greatly enriched by a stop.

During the peak tourist season, roughly from late March through early November, visitor center hours are 8 A.M.– 9 P.M. Winter hours are 8 A.M.–5 P.M. Evening programs at South Campground's Amphitheater and naturalist programs at the visitor center are conducted from spring through fall. Children's programs are conducted twice daily at the nature center, near the campground amphitheater, from Memorial Day through Labor Day. Parents can leave their children here and enjoy a short hike in the canyon.

Ranger-guided hikes include Riverside Walk; up the Narrows to Orderville Canyon; Angels Landing; the Emerald Pools Trail to Middle Pool;

the Watchman Trail; the Canyon Overlook Trail; and naturalists-choice hikes.

Springdale, Utah, located at the mouth of Zion Canyon just south of the park's south entrance, offers a full line of services for park visitors. Hikers, however, are advised to come prepared, since there is little hiking equipment available in town. Springdale has several motels, restaurants, gas stations, and grocery stores. The communities of St. George, Hurricane, Kanab, and Cedar City also have a wide array of services and accommodations. Hospitals are located in St. George, Kanab, and Cedar City.

Campgrounds

The private Zion Canyon Campground, a short distance south of the South Entrance, offers a spacious, shady campground with tent sites and full hookups for RVs. Hot showers, a laundry, and a market are also available.

Zion has two large public campgrounds, one of which remains open through the winter. Watchman and South campgrounds are located a short distance north of the South Entrance. Overnight camping fees are collected at the self-registration station at each campground.

Watchman Campground is Zion's largest, with 246 campsites on a bench above North Fork Virgin River at 3900 feet. Young boxelders, velvet ash, netleaf hackberry, and Fremont cottonwoods shade campers, but are still small enough to allow fine views of the canyon walls, including the fluted cliffs of The Watchman and Bridge Mountain. South Campground, at 3950 feet, is considerably smaller, with 141 campsites. Large netleaf hackberry and Fremont cottonwoods provide ample shade for campers at this pleasant riverside campground. These two campgrounds often fill by early- to mid-afternoon during the spring-through-fall peak season, so come early if you plan to camp here.

Lava Point Campground is a stark contrast to the desert-like campgrounds in Zion Canyon. It rests atop the lava-capped mesa of Lava Point at 7900 feet. This is a primitive campground, and since no water is provided, no fee is charged. Its six campsites are shaded by white fir, ponderosa pine, aspen, and Gambel oak. Views from the campsites are limited to the peaceful forest that surrounds it.

Wood gathering in the park is prohibited, so if you want to build a fire in the grills provided at each campground, bring your own.

Zion has two developed picnic sites. The Grotto Picnic Area is on the shady canyon floor between Red Arch Mountain and The Spearhead. A large parking area serves the spacious picnic area, at 4290 feet. The Kolob Canyons Viewpoint (elevation 6300 feet) at the roadend in the Kolob section of Zion also boasts a small but delightful picnic area. Nestled against a hillside in a woodland of pinyon and juniper, this site offers some of the most dramatic views in all of the park.

Visitors are free to picnic wherever they wish in the park, but all should be sure to pack out all their trash, including orange and banana peels—these "biodegradable" items will not decompose in the arid desert climate.

Zion Lodge offers a variety of services and accommodations. A motel, motel suites, and western cabins are available for an overnight stay, but guests are advised to make reservations four to six months in advance. The lodge is open all year. A restaurant and a gift shop are here. Guided tram tours are available, and arrangements for horseback rides along the Sand Bench Trail and information on the shuttle service for hikers are also available at Zion Lodge.

For further information:

Park information:
Park Superintendent
Zion National Park
Springdale, UT 84767
(435) 772-3256
www.nps.gov/zion
For shuttle information: (435) 772-0312

Information regarding the private Zion Canyon Campground:
Zion Canyon Campground
P.O. Box 99
Springdale, UT 84767
(435) 772-3237

Information regarding Zion Lodge:
TW Services, Inc.
P.O. Box 400
Cedar City, UT 84721
(435) 586-7686 (individuals) or
(435) 586-7624 (groups)

Hiking in Zion

The trail network of Zion National Park provides a wide array of hiking opportunities to satisfy anyone wishing to park the car and experience this magnificent landscape at a leisurely pace. Ranging from paved 5-minute strolls to backpack trips of several days, Zion's more than 100 miles of trails sample virtually every aspect of the park. But you need not be a dedicated backpacker to enjoy the majesty of Zion. The hikes described below range from 30-minute walks to half-day hikes that visit some of Zion's highlights and sample a wide range of memorable landscapes.

Zion's trails claim more than 5000 feet of vertical relief, and boast scenery that includes vast plateaus clad in pine, fir, and aspen; deep and narrow canyons that lie in eternal shadow; sun-baked expanses of open desert; lofty vista points; pinyon-juniper woodlands; and the green spreads of lava-rimmed meadows.

As does the scenery, the trails themselves vary greatly. Some are faint paths seldom trod by park visitors, while others are paved and frequently used. Some of Zion's shorter paved trails offer access to wheelchairs and even baby strollers. There are cliff-hanging trails that are intermittently paved where they were blasted into steep cliffs of Navajo Sandstone, providing sure footing on what otherwise would be a sandy, slippery, dangerous trail.

Common-sense rules of desert hiking apply in the backcountry of this diverse park, as they do for hiking elsewhere on the Colorado Plateau. Lightning, flash floods, rockfall, and dehydration, to name but a few hazards, are always possible and should not be taken lightly (see the chapter "Hiking Utah's Desert Parks"). Novice hikers who may be uncomfortable hiking the trails on their own, and anyone wishing to gain a better appreciation of the natural history of the park, can take advantage of naturalist-led hikes on many of Zion's shorter trails. Schedules of guided hikes are posted at the Zion Canyon visitor center.

Weather in Zion, though often pleasant, can range from extremes of heat and drought to bitter cold, snow and severe thunderstorms. Annual precipitation ranges from an estimated 21 inches atop the plateaus to 15 inches in Zion Canyon, and recorded temperature extremes range from 115° to 15° below zero. Two pronounced wet seasons occur in Zion, the first from winter to early spring, and the second, dominated by thunderstorms, from mid to late summer. Each season in Zion is as distinctive as it is beautiful. Whatever time of year you visit the park, you are sure to return home filled with vivid memories of a unique landscape.

The Zion Canyon transportation system

In recent years, parking areas at trailheads in Zion Canyon have been filled to capacity every day during the peak season, forcing some visitors to abandon their plans for hiking the trails of the canyon. Since many visitors spend only a day or two in the park, that congestion has ruined many vacations. To alleviate congestion and gridlock in Zion Canyon during the season of peak use, the Zion Canyon Transportation System was implemented in the spring of 2000. The system ensures that visitors will be able to reach their chosen trailhead while they sit back and relax in a shuttle bus, soaking in the scenery instead of watching out for traffic and pedestrians while searching for a parking place.

Between late March and late October, the first half of the Scenic Drive from Canyon Junction to Zion Lodge will be open only to hikers, bicyclists, shuttle vehicles, private vehicles of overnight lodge guests, and Zion Lodge tour buses. From the lodge to the road's end at Temple of Sinawava, use will be restricted to hikers, bicyclists, and shuttle buses. Shuttle buses will offer access to the following stops on the Scenic Drive: Canyon Junction, Court of the Patriarchs, Zion Lodge, Grotto Picnic Area, Weeping Rock, Big Bend, and Temple of Sinawava. The Scenic Drive will be open to private vehicles during the remainder of the year.

Visitors staying in or near Springdale can access the shuttle buses at several developed shuttle stops. Park visitors can access the shuttle system from the visitor center/transit center adjacent to Watchman Campground. Contact Zion National Park for more information. ■

Hike 1. Watchman Trail

Distance	2.9 miles semiloop trip
Elevation gain	500'
Average hiking time	1½ hours
Difficulty rating	3
Child rating	2
Best season	Open all year, but very hot in summer and possibly snow-covered in winter.
Hazards	Steep dropoffs near the trail's end.

Driving to the trailhead

To reach Zion National Park, follow the directions below.

If you are traveling from the south via Interstate 15, take the Utah Highway 9 exit, 10 miles north of St. George, which is signed for Zion National Park, and proceed 11 miles through the town of Hurricane to La Verkin. From the north, take the Toquerville exit off Interstate 15 and drive southeast on Utah 17 for 6 miles to La Verkin and the junction with Utah 9.

Drive east from La Verkin on Utah Highway 9 for 19.9 miles to the South Entrance of Zion National Park. Immediately beyond the entrance station, turn right (east) onto the road signed for the entrance to Watchman Campground and the visitor center, bridge the North Fork Virgin River, and soon come to the spacious parking lot at the visitor center, 0.2 mile east of Utah Highway 9.

Visitors approaching from the east via U.S. Highway 89 should turn west onto Utah 9 at Mt. Carmel Junction, 18 miles northwest of Kanab, and 127 miles south of Richfield. Follow Utah 9 west for 24.6 miles to the junction with the Zion Canyon Scenic Drive, turn left (south), and proceed 0.8 mile to the Watchman Campground/visitor center turnoff. The large parking lot at the visitor center lies 0.2 mile east of the turnoff.

Introduction

The Watchman Trail is a short but scenic route leading to a rocky bench on the east slopes of lower Zion Canyon, offering unique vistas available from no other trail in the park. The bench lies below a prominent red spire rising 2500 feet from the canyon floor, dubbed The Watchman by early Mormon settlers. The trail is a fine leg-stretcher for guests of Zion Canyon's campgrounds, and its unique views and interesting terrain make the trip a good choice for the hiker with limited time and energy.

Description

Hikers can begin this trip from either of two points: the visitor center parking lot, or your campsite in Watchman Campground. The signed trailhead (3900') is located on the north side of the visitor center/Watchman Campground access road, immediately north of the transportation-center shuttle-bus shelter. From the trailhead the trail proceeds northeast across a terrace between the North Fork Virgin River and the paved access road to ranger residences. We head northeast across the flat grass- and rabbitbrush-covered terrace, reaching the residence access road after 0.25 mile, which we cross and then resume our trail walk on the opposite side. After leaving the road, pause long enough to gaze northeast up to imposing Bridge Mountain, rearing 2800 feet above us. Those with sharp eyesight or with binoculars can make out a narrow stone arch on the skyline north of the peak. A host of jagged summits form the rugged skyline above us, from Bridge Mountain in the northeast to Johnson Mountain at Zion Canyon's mouth.

Our trail presently takes us across a wide bench, studded with four-wing saltbush, opposite a group of park employee residences. From here the trail heads east up a minor canyon and begins ascending beneath imposing cliffs. Our trail takes us upward through the varicolored mudstones and siltstones of the Dinosaur Canyon layer of the Moenave Formation. Proceeding upward toward the next layer in that formation, the Springdale Sandstone, we'll notice undercut ledges created by the differential erosion of a soft rock layer underlying a harder, more resistant one.

After negotiating four switchbacks, we curve into the head of the canyon, where several sluggish springs host lush riparian vegetation, such as Fremont cottonwood, boxelder, and a variety of seasonal wildflowers. These springs give life to the small, seasonal stream that trickles into the canyon below. Ahead we begin a southwestward traverse while enjoying increasingly outstanding vistas from the north-facing canyon wall. Here we notice a change in vegetation, for a comparatively cooler microclimate prevails on this more sheltered slope. Utah juniper and now singleleaf pinyon predominate among shrubs typical of the pinyon-juniper woodland, such as buffaloberry, singleleaf ash, Utah serviceberry, and yucca.

Where it attains the high bench above Zion Canyon, the trail forks after 1.25 miles, forming a scenic loop around the perimeter of the bench. Hikers eager to enjoy unobstructed vistas will bear right for now, returning via the left fork. The trail winds along the Springdale Sandstone-capped rim, soon reaching a junction. A spur to an overlook forks to the right here, quickly leading to the brink of the rim at 4420 feet, where a broad panorama unfolds.

Below, at the wide mouth of Zion Canyon, is the town of Springdale, a Mormon settlement dating back to the 1860s. Beyond the town are the aptly named Vermilion Cliffs, adorned by the landmark Eagle Crags. Those rugged cliffs, composed of Moenave Formation rocks, the same rocks as those upon which we stand, are one of the "risers" forming southern Utah's Grand Staircase.

Towers of the Virgin rear mightily toward the heavens across the wide floor of Zion Canyon, boasting a vertical relief of nearly 4000 feet. Our view also extends up the narrowing canyon, encompassing a myriad of colorful, soaring cliffs, crags, and tree-topped plateaus. To return via the loop trail, backtrack from the overlook and turn right. This longer side of the loop follows the rim of the bench eastward, then turns abruptly northwest, where we climb easily amid sandstone blocks, pinyon, juniper, and various shrubs, soon reaching the main trail after another 0.4 mile, where we bear right to retrace our route for 1.25 miles to the trailhead. ■

Hike 2. Emerald Pools Trail

Distance	2.1 miles loop trip
Elevation gain	320'
Average hiking time	1 hour
Difficulty rating	2
Child rating	2
Best season	All year
Hazards	Steep dropoffs; avoid when ice- or snow-covered.

Driving to the trailhead

Follow the driving directions for Hike 1 to reach the Zion Canyon visitor center. From mid-May through October you must board a shuttle bus at the transit center adjacent to the new visitor center. Ride the shuttle bus to the bus stop at Zion Lodge, and disembark there.

At other times of the year you may drive your private vehicle to the trailhead. From Canyon Junction (the junction of Utah 9 and Zion Canyon Scenic Drive), 1.7 miles north of the visitor center, drive north on the Scenic Drive for 2.6 miles to the spacious trailhead parking area, signed for EMERALD POOLS and HORSE CORRAL, on the left (west) side of the road.

Introduction

This very scenic one-hour jaunt is one of Zion Canyon's most-used trails. It tours a shady side canyon featuring a perennial stream with dense vegetation and four limpid pools reflecting towering canyon walls. Hikers not inclined to undertake the entire loop can follow the mile-long paved trail (accessible to wheelchairs) to the lower pool and a dripping alcove resplendent with water-loving vegetation.

Description

From the shuttle-bus stop at Zion Lodge, cross the lodge grounds to the Scenic Drive, where you will find the trailhead immediately to the west (4280'), signed for EMERALD POOLS and HORSE CORRAL. The signed trail quickly bridges North Fork Virgin River west of the large parking area, then immediately forks. The right fork, a gently climbing, paved trail, offers the shortest and easiest route to the lower pool, while the left fork offers access to the loop trail and to a riverside spur trail leading to the Sand Bench Trail.

Turning left beneath the soaring heights of Lady Mountain, we stroll south along the shady riverbank, under the spreading branches of Fremont cottonwood, water birch, and Gambel oak. Quite soon we reach a signed junction at 0.1 mile, where the riverside stock trail (also open to hikers) continues down-river and the loop trail climbs the slope above.

At the junction, we turn right, and a single switchback ensues, followed by a protracted traverse. The trail quickly crosses slide debris beneath Lady Mountain, a soaring crag rising 2500 feet above the trail. Shrub live oak, Utah juniper, Gambel oak, singleleaf pinyon, Utah serviceberry, buffaloberry, singleleaf ash, narrowleaf yucca, and prickly pear are thickly massed along the mountainside above the canyons. Enroute we'll splash through the runoff of several verdant springs, their courses banked with cottonwood, water birch, and boxelder.

Views throughout the traverse are inspiring, encompassing square-edged mesas topped with tall pines, sculptured cliffs streaked with curtains of red, and the gaping cleft of Zion Canyon. The trail maintains a gentle grade, and is intermittently paved above steep dropoffs.

As the trail curves around a shoulder of the slope, the manicured grounds of Zion Lodge come into view, and several outstanding landmarks form a ragged skyline above the canyon. Among them, from north to south, are Angels Landing, The Great White Throne, Mountain of the Sun, and Twin Brothers. The prominent gothic arch on the flanks of imposing Red Arch Mountain, just south of The Great White Throne, was formed in 1880 when an enormous slab of Navajo Sandstone spalled off the cliff and buried Mormon pioneer Oliver D. Gifford's cornfield. Altogether, the peaceful floor of Zion Canyon, with the river threading its way among grassy openings and groves of cottonwoods, and with a backdrop of soaring sandstone cliffs, makes a most attractive picture.

As the trail enters the Heaps Canyon drainage, we are confronted by a gigantic amphitheater, its north wall of Navajo Sandstone intricately cross-bedded and capped by the prominent spire of The Spearhead. Below us, the perennial waters of the canyon nourish a dense forest of Gambel oak, boxelder, and Fremont cottonwood.

Where more springs course over the trail ahead, bigtooth maples arch their branches overhead, their leaves turning a brilliant red after the first frosts of autumn. As we approach the draw of the canyon, Douglas-firs appear on trailside slopes, and soon Heaps Canyon creek comes into view, pouring off an overhanging ledge between the middle and lower pools. Immediately below the overhang, a seepline nurtures a narrow strip of hanging gardens.

Soon we reach middle Emerald Pool at 0.9 mile, perched near the brink of the pouroff and rimmed by Douglas-firs, willows, Utah junipers, and Fremont cottonwoods. The small, still pool reflects an exciting backdrop of

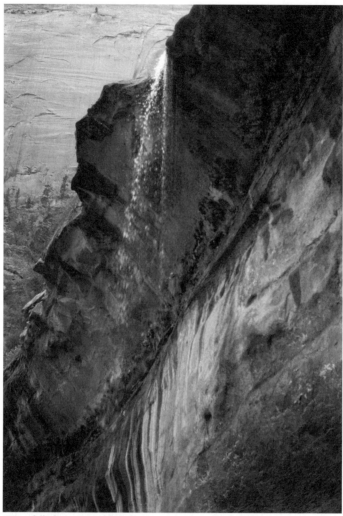

Waterfall above Emerald Pools

sculptured, pastel-shaded canyon walls. Overhead, tall ponderosa pines form scattered silhouette figures atop the canyon rim.

Proceeding 50 yards beyond the pool to a junction, we ponder the option of turning left and ascending to the upper pool or turning right and looping back to the trailhead. The upper pool is the largest and deepest, and well worth a visit. The trail leading to it crosses a slope littered with boulders that were spread across the trail by a major flash flood in 1987. The correct route may be lost amid a confusing array of use trails, all of which ultimately lead to the upper pool.

As we ascend the brushy slope at a moderately steep grade, an abundance of creeping hollygrape at the trail's edge heralds our approach to the upper pool, where the grade abates. Quite soon we reach the edge of the large pool at 1.1 miles (4600'), where velvet ash, willow, bigtooth maple, and boxelder, many of them draped by vines of the canyon wild grape, crowd the edge and provide a shady canopy for hikers on a hot day.

Numerous springs and seeps feed the pool, and after heavy rains or the melting of the snowpack on the plateau above, a noisy waterfall plunges over the tall cliff behind the pool. Rising sheer above us on three sides are lofty cliffs of Navajo Sandstone, stained with desert varnish from dust and mineral-laden rainwater. Notice the Douglas-firs clinging to the ledges on the cliff face south of the pool. That north-facing cliff is shaded from heat and sunlight, so soil moisture evaporates more slowly and nurtures a suitable microhabitat for trees that are more commonly found atop the plateaus more than 3000 feet above.

After backtracking for 0.2 mile to the junction near the middle pool, we should bear left if we intend to complete the circuit. Quickly we meet a left-branching trail bound for the Grotto Picnic Area, 0.8 mile ahead. But we turn right, passing through a narrow cleft between two immense boulders fallen from the cliffs above. Rock stairs then lower us for 0.1 mile to a junction with another left-branching trail, which quickly connects with the aforementioned trail leading to the picnic area.

Our trail immediately leads us under an overhanging ledge just above the lower pool, which is merely a wide spot in the creekbed. Presently wedged between the cliff face and the waterfall emanating from the middle pool, our wet trail leads us past horizontal seeplines resplendent with the growth of hanging gardens. A white, powdery residue of sodium bicarbonate coats the trailside wall, left behind by the evaporation of seeping water. We are likely to get wet under the dripping wall as we proceed out of the canyon's draw and begin the final leg of the loop. The trail presently traverses southeast across lower slopes of the amphitheater beneath a canopy of Gambel oak and bigtooth maple, their ranks mixed with Utah juniper and singleleaf ash. Inspiring views of canyons, cliffs, and mesa rims accompany us as we descend to the floor of Zion Canyon. Reaching the river, the trail hugs the west bank the remaining distance to the bridge, from where we quickly backtrack to the parking area, 0.7 mile from the last junction. ■

Hike 3. West Rim Trail: Grotto Picnic Area to Scout Lookout and Angels Landing

Distance	3.8 miles round trip to Scout Lookout; 4.8 miles round trip to Angels Landing
Elevation gain	1060' to Scout Lookout; 1500' to Angels Landing
Average hiking times	2 to 2½ hours to Scout Lookout; 2½ to 3 hours to Angels Landing
Difficulty rating	4 to 5
Child rating	3
Best season	March through November
Hazards	Steep dropoffs; avoid when snow- or ice-covered or when a thunderstorm is threatening.

Driving to the trailhead

Follow the driving directions for Hike 1 to reach the Zion Canyon visitor center. From mid-May through October you must board a shuttle bus at the transit center adjacent to the new visitor center. Ride the shuttle bus to the bus stop at Grotto Picnic Area, and disembark there.

At other times of the year you may drive your private vehicle to the trailhead. From Canyon Junction (the junction of Utah 9 and Zion Canyon Scenic Drive), 1.7 miles north of the visitor center, drive north on the Scenic Drive for 3.4 miles to the spacious trailhead parking area, opposite the Grotto Picnic Area, on the left (west) side of the road.

Introduction

The highly scenic trail to Scout Lookout, built in 1926, was among the first to be constructed in Zion. One section of the trail, a series of switchbacks called Walter's Wiggles, is an engineering marvel, spanning an otherwise impassable cliff to allow access to a memorable viewpoint 1000 feet above the floor of Zion Canyon.

The route to Angels Landing from Scout Lookout is rigorous and exposed, in places requiring the use of both hands and feet. Faint-hearted hikers and small children should not attempt this steep trail. It's a dangerous route even during fair weather, and only the foolhardy will attempt it when it is snow- or ice-covered, or when a thunderstorm is threatening. Both trails receive moderate use.

Description

From the Grotto trailhead parking area/shuttle-bus stop (4290'), we immediately cross the river via a bridge. A pleasant riverside stroll ensues, leading to a moderate ascent upon brushy slopes, amid a jumble of boulders from a Cathedral Mountain rockslide.

Paved switchbacks carved into the Navajo Sandstone elevate us into the shady, narrow hanging gorge of Refrigerator Canyon. A pleasant stroll along the floor of the cliff-framed chasm, a delightful spot to rest on a hot day, leads us to more switchbacks. Ascending the 250-foot wall above the canyon, we negotiate Walter's Wiggles, above which we step out onto the canyon rim amid scattered ponderosa pines.

Nearby, a sign identifies Scout Lookout, at 1.9 miles (5350'). Many day-hikers terminate their journey here, satisfied with the superb views into Zion Canyon directly below, and east into the gaping alcove at the mouth of precipitous Echo Canyon, flanked on either side by majestic, soaring cliffs.

• • • • • • • • • • • •

Angels Landing

The sentinel monolith of Angels Landing juts outward into Zion Canyon, forcing the south-flowing river to make a great bend around it and its lower satellite rock, The Organ. Hikers with a fear of heights should be content with the exceptional views from Scout Lookout and avoid the Angels Landing Trail.

From the signed junction immediately below Scout Lookout the trail follows the pine-clad rim generally south, climbing over a minor rise before attacking the north ridge of the landing. The route, cut into solid rock, very steeply ascends a knife-edged sandstone rib, from which cliffs plunge 500 feet or more on either side. Sloping steps cut into the rock make footing precarious. Intermittent segments of chain bolted to the rock offer occasional handholds, but many exposed stretches offer no such protection. The route is steepest and most exposed just below the top, but once we surmount the crest we simply follow the narrow ridge among scattered ponderosa pines to the high point on the canyon rim (5790'), 0.5 mile from Scout Lookout, where an incredible, aerial-like view unfolds.

Seemingly a stone's throw away across the gaping maw of Zion Canyon is the park's most famous landmark, The Great White Throne. Rivaling some of the world's greatest stone monoliths in size, form, and relief, its sheer cliffs rear abruptly 2200 feet from the canyon to the broad mesa above. Also capturing our attention is the 1000-foot red-stained wall of Cable Mountain. The wooden frame of the Draw Works, constructed by ingenious pioneers to transport lumber from the plateau to the canyon bottom, is visible along the edge of that mountain. The trail leading to Cable Mountain and Observation Point can be visually traced along the canyon wall as it climbs above the verdant growth engulfing Weeping Rock. Fine cliff-framed views extend southward down Zion Canyon, and North Fork Virgin River is not only seen but heard.

Retrace your steps with caution back to the Grotto trailhead. ■

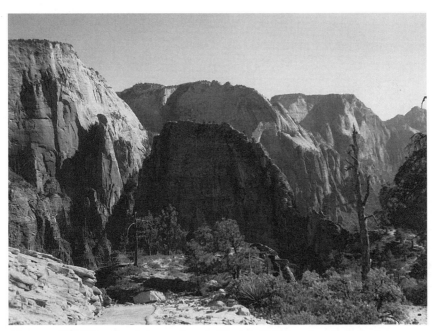

The great cliffs of Zion Canyon as seen from the West Rim Trail just above Scout Lookout; Angels Landing rises at center

Hike 4. Weeping Rock to Hidden Canyon

Distance	2.2 miles round trip
Elevation gain	750′
Average hiking time	1½ hours
Difficulty rating	3
Child rating	3
Best season	March through November
Hazards	Steep dropoffs, little shade; trail should be avoided if thunderstorms threaten. Snow or ice makes travel hazardous from late fall through early spring.

Driving to the trailhead

Follow the driving directions for Hike 1 to reach the Zion Canyon visitor center. From mid-May through October you must board a shuttle bus at the transit center adjacent to the new visitor center. Ride the shuttle bus to the bus stop at Weeping Rock, and disembark there.

At other times of the year you may drive your private vehicle to the trailhead. From Canyon Junction (the junction of Utah 9 and Zion Canyon Scenic Drive), 1.7 miles north of the visitor center, drive north on the Scenic Drive for 4.6 miles to the spacious trailhead parking area at Weeping Rock.

Introduction

This exceptionally scenic trip leads into the narrow hanging gorge of Hidden Canyon, a pleasant retreat on a hot day. The general route of the trail dates back to the time when Native Americans inhabited the region, offering them access to the plateaus for hunting and gathering forays. Later, the trail was improved upon by pioneers driving cattle to summer range. The Flanigan brothers used the route while developing their cable draw works on Cable Mountain.

Description

From the Weeping Rock parking area (4350'), we follow the Observation Point Trail as it bridges Echo Canyon creek and bear right where the Weeping Rock Trail forks left. We quickly exit the narrow ribbon of riparian growth hugging the streambank, climbing steeply at once upon rubbly slide debris. Above this slope we reach concrete pavement and begin ascending a series of moderately steep switchbacks cut into the cliff face beneath the seemingly overhanging wall of Cable Mountain. Views enroute stretch across Zion Canyon to the sentinel rock of Angels Landing.

At the eighth switchback, the signed trail to Hidden Canyon peels off to the right at 0.6 mile and 4850 feet, and from here we have a fine view back down to the shady alcove of Weeping Rock. Turning right onto that unpaved trail, we begin switchbacking at a moderate grade amid pines and firs, directly beneath the sheer walls of Cable Mountain. Above this climb, a traverse leads us into a shady chasm supporting Douglas-fir, white fir, ponderosa pine, and velvet ash. Soon the trail exits the chasm via a low but slippery slickrock wall, where acrophobic hikers may be compelled to turn back.

Beyond that traverse, we curve into the mouth of Hidden Canyon, hanging 700 feet above the floor of Zion Canyon. Numerous potholes have been worn into the Navajo Sandstone slickrock floor of the canyon by abrasive runoff waters. These waterpockets are like those commonly encountered in the same rock unit in Capitol Reef National Park, and they may hold water after substantial rains.

Steps cut into the rock allow passage around some of the potholes, but soon we are forced into the narrow, sandy, rocky wash as giant cliffs close in on either side. The trail apparently ends where we dip into the wash at 1.1 miles (5180'), and some hikers may be content to go this far, but to others, this mysterious chasm beckons. Douglas-fir, white fir, and ponderosa pine thrive in this relatively cool, moist microclimate within the confines of the canyon. Great sheer cliffs soar heavenward on either side of the narrow, arrow-straight canyon. A number of small alcoves and other erosional features await those who hike the dry wash upstream, for another 0.5 mile or so. Rock climbing skills are necessary to reach the head of the canyon. ■

Hike 5. Riverside Walk, Orderville Canyon

Distance	2.0 miles round trip to the trail's end; 6.4 miles, round trip to mouth of Orderville Canyon
Elevation gain	70' for Riverside Walk; 200' to reach the mouth of Orderville Canyon
Average hiking times	1 hour for Riverside Walk; 3½ to 4 hours for Orderville Canyon
Difficulty rating	1 for Riverside Walk; 4 for Orderville Canyon
Child rating	1 for Riverside Walk; 3 for Orderville Canyon
Best season	Trail open all year, but may be snow-covered at times during winter. River hiking is best from May through September.
Hazards	Negligible along trail; deep wading beyond trail's end over a slippery river bottom, and the possibility of flash floods and cold water. Check on river and weather conditions at the park visitor center.

Driving to the trailhead

Follow the driving directions for Hike 1 to reach the Zion Canyon visitor center. From mid-May through October you must board a shuttle bus at the transit center adjacent to the new visitor center. Ride the shuttle bus to the end of the road at Temple of Sinawava, and disembark there.

At other times of the year you may drive your private vehicle to the trailhead. From Canyon Junction (the junction of Utah 9 and Zion Canyon Scenic Drive), 1.7 miles north of the visitor center, drive north on the Scenic Drive for 6.2 miles to the spacious Temple of Sinawava trailhead parking area at the end of the road.

Introduction

Riverside Walk is Zion's most heavily used trail, and with good reason. Seeping alcoves, luxurious hanging gardens, shady riparian woodlands, a nearly level trail (paved for wheelchair access), and an ever-narrowing and ever-deepening canyon draw visitors from the world over. Many hike beyond the trail's end into The Narrows, one of the classic canyon treks on the Colorado Plateau.

Slicing into the heart of the Markagunt Plateau, the North Fork Virgin River has carved a canyon 1000-2000 feet deep, and ranging in width from 200 yards at the Temple of Sinawava to barely 20 feet above Orderville Canyon.

To negotiate any part of The Narrows beyond the trail, hikers must be well prepared, and must not underestimate the hazards of wading through a knee-deep river in a narrow flash-flood-prone canyon. Few trips in Zion are more rewarding, or potentially more dangerous, than wading the Virgin River through The Narrows on a hot, clear summer day. But forays into the canyon from the Temple of Sinawava are for dayhiking only. Flash flood danger can make this hike life-threatening. Each hiker is responsible for obtaining updated information on river conditions and weather forecasts from the visitor center, and all are responsible for their personal safety.

Never hike into The Narrows alone, and be sure to have a sturdy staff for balance and lightweight, rubber-soled shoes for traction on the slippery river bottom. Hikers can obtain a pamphlet at the park visitor center explaining the hazards and precautions one should take before entering the canyon.

Description

Since this trail is the park's most popular, expect plenty of company as you stroll up the trail beyond the parking area (4418'), flanked by the redrock tower of the Temple of Sinawava on one side and the unimposing red spire of The Pulpit on the other. The trail leads upstream, east of the river, in the shadow of tall, broken cliffs. White fir and Douglas-fir stand tall on the canyon walls above us, while the canyon floor is well-shaded by velvet ash and boxelder. Along the way we'll pass interpretive signs explaining canyon widening, hanging gardens (where the Zion rock snail, a species endemic to The Narrows, makes its home), a rockslide, and a perpetually wet desert swamp. Many visitors enjoy picnicking along the rushing river, and some of them may wish to follow a use trail that goes left only 100 yards from the trailhead, quickly leading to the river's edge.

The trail ends where the canyon bends northeast at 1.0 mile (4490'), and hikers unprepared for river hiking are advised to go no farther. But those who are prepared simply plunge into the river, either crossing to the opposite bank or following its waters upstream. The river is usually only knee-deep, but depending on recent rains or snowmelt runoff, it can be much deeper, and swift. Even during low water, expect some holes to be waist-deep or even deeper. Use your staff to probe deep holes as you proceed.

The canyon becomes increasingly narrow, and even in summer, little sunlight penetrates into this narrow corridor. Boxelder grows on riverside benches in tandem with white fir, a tree typically found on the plateaus 3000 feet above. The river meanders below Orderville Canyon; along this stretch we can crisscross it between sandy benches, following short trails between crossings.

Mystery Falls, a 100-foot cascade backdropped by rugged Mountain of Mystery, is the first of many outstanding features we encounter along the way. We pass numerous springs and seeps nurturing verdant hanging gardens that decorate fluted canyon walls stained with streaks of red and dark patches of desert varnish.

As we proceed, we should choose our crossings carefully, as the riverbed is strewn with slippery, moss-covered rocks. Black basalt rocks and boulders, from the plateaus far above, are abundant and particularly slick. Approaching Orderville Canyon we are forced into the river more frequently, as the benches are fewer and more widely spaced. Orderville Canyon contributes its small stream to the river at 3.2 miles (4620') where it exits a narrow cleft on our right (east).

On the return trip, wade the river with care. ■

Hike 6. Canyon Overlook Trail

Distance	1.0 mile round trip
Elevation gain	110'
Average hiking time	30 minutes
Difficulty rating	2
Child rating	2
Best season	All year, but the trail should be avoided when ice- or snow-covered, or if thunderstorms threaten.
Hazards	Steep dropoffs; no shade.

Driving to the trailhead

Hikers Driving to Zion from the west should follow the driving directions for Hike 1 to reach the Zion Canyon visitor center. From there follow Utah 9 north for 1.7 miles to Canyon Junction, and then bear right, staying on Utah 9. At the eastern portal of the Zion-Mt. Carmel Tunnel, 4.5 miles from Zion Canyon, park in the parking area on the southeast side of the road.

Hikers approaching from U.S. 89 on the east will follow Utah 9 west from Mt. Carmel Junction for 20 miles to the trailhead.

Introduction

This short, self-guided nature trail leads across slickrock to a grand vista point high above Pine Creek canyon. Views into lower Zion Canyon, 1000 feet below, include some of the most striking landmarks in the park. The hike should appeal to hikers of varied abilities, and is an especially fine choice for a short stroll if one has limited time or energy.

An interpretive leaflet available at the trailhead or the visitor center explains the natural history of the area, and should help hikers to gain knowledge and better appreciate what they encounter along the trail.

Ranger-led walks are frequently conducted on this trail; check the schedule of interpretive activities at the visitor center.

Description

From the parking area at the east portal of the Zion-Mt. Carmel Tunnel, carefully cross the highway to the beginning of the trail (5130'), indicated by a small sign. A series of steps soon leads to a traverse high above the narrow cleft of Pine Creek canyon. Despite the presence of handrails along exposed stretches, hikers should nonetheless exercise caution throughout the trail's length.

A variety of seasonal wildflowers adorn the Navajo Sandstone slickrock among such trailside shrubs as squawbush, buffaloberry, singleleaf ash, and shrub live oak, and an occasional Utah juniper.

Where we curve into a prominent but narrow side canyon, maidenhair fern appears in the moist and sheltered habitat beneath an overhanging slab. Other denizens of these rocky environs include singleleaf pinyon, littleleaf mountain mahogany (found exclusively on and near slickrock), and Utah serviceberry. Ahead we encounter more maidenhair fern, growing along a seepline that dampens the wall of a trailside alcove.

Upon exiting the side canyon, we continue to follow the seepline, and soon pass a lone Fremont cottonwood, further evidence of ample moisture within the sandstone. The slickrock trail ahead winds among tilted sandstone slabs, soon reaching a fenced overlook at 0.5 mile (5255'), perched on the rim above Pine Creek canyon. The Great Arch, that deep, arch-shaped alcove seen from the highway below, invisible from our vantage, lies just below the brink of the cliff. Thousand-foot slopes plunging from Bridge Mountain and East Temple frame a stirring view of the Towers of the Virgin, a host of rugged crags rising nearly 4000 feet above the canyon floor. A plaque at the overlook identifies many of the prominent landmarks that meet our gaze.

One of the five galleries in the Zion-Mt. Carmel Tunnel can be seen on the cliff below. During the three years of construction in the late 1920s, narrow-gauge rail cars hauled waste rock from the tunnel to the galleries, from where it was dumped over the cliff into Pine Creek canyon.

Above us, conspicuous cross-bedding on the face of the Navajo Sandstone, formed as ancient winds swept across a vast sand desert, offer evidence that the world has not always been the same as it is today.

Return the way you came. ■

Hike 7. Pine Valley to Northgate Peaks Overlook

Distance	5 miles round trip
Elevation gain	50'
Average hiking time	2½ hours
Difficulty rating	3
Child rating	2 to 3
Best season	May through October
Hazards	Negligible

Driving to the trailhead

From the town of Virgin on Utah 9, 6.1 miles east of La Verkin and 14.1 miles west of the South Entrance to Zion, follow the paved Kolob Terrace Road generally northeast for 15.3 miles to the signed Wildcat Canyon Trailhead spur road, branching right (south). Follow this narrow, unpaved spur south for 0.1 mile to the trailhead on the edge of spacious Pine Valley.

Introduction

This scenic trip leads the hiker from the lava rimrock of the Kolob Terrace to the sandstone realm of lofty domes and crags at the Northgate Peaks Overlook. The moderately used trail features oak-rimmed meadows, peaceful, park-like forests of ponderosa pine, and far-ranging vistas.

Description

The Wildcat Canyon Trail begins at the Pine Valley Trailhead (7000'), beneath the 7415-foot dome of Pine Valley Peak. The trail, rocky at first, heads east along the fringe of a charred grove of Gambel oak, where silky lupine and Palmer penstemon grow in profusion at the trailside. After rising gradually, we begin an almost imperceptible downgrade leading through the park-like stands of ponderosa pine in Pine Valley.

After 1.2 miles, we cross a shallow, usually dry wash, and immediately thereafter reach a junction with the so-called Connector Trail, heading generally west for 4 miles to the Hop Valley Trailhead on the Kolob Terrace Road. Bear left at the junction and ascend the rocky trail eastward for about 250 yards to the Northgate Peaks Trail, and turn right (south).

The Northgate Peaks Trail, sandy in places, follows the nearly level plateau south through a lovely forest of ponderosa pine. The trail splits after 125 yards, with the left (southeast) fork leading to a cairned route that descends the head of Russell Gulch, affording a route to The Subway for

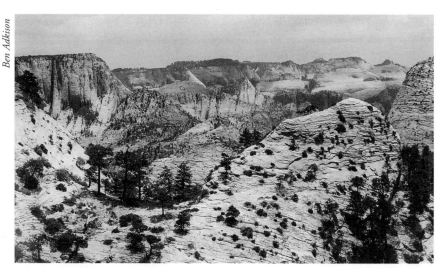

Ben Adkison

View southeast from Northgate Peaks

experienced canyoneers only. A sign at the junction details permit requirements for Subway hikers.

Taking the right fork, we gain little elevation, and before long we reach the basalt-capped overlook at 2.5 miles (6900'), perched on a point of the plateau, with the slickrock domes of Northgate Peaks flanking us on either side. The incredible view that unfolds is well worth the effort required to get here.

The gargantuan dome of 7395-foot North Guardian Angel dominates our southward view over the labyrinth of rugged canyons draining Left Fork North Creek. On the far southern horizon, framed between North Guardian Angel and west Northgate Peak, the domes of Mounts Trumbull and Logan punctuate the Shivwits Plateau in northwest Arizona. Russell Gulch, the slickrock-bound gorge below to the east, is a challenging route used by experienced canyoneers, with a permit, to gain access to Left Fork North Creek and The Subway.

A host of striking cliffs, crags, buttes, and mesas meets our gaze as we look southeast, but towering above them all toward the south is the lofty platform of West Temple. As we face west, the distant hogback crest of the 10,000-foot Pine Valley Mountains is framed by the sandstone domes of the western Northgate Peak and Pine Valley Peak.

One can't help but notice the prominent cross-bedding on virtually all of the nearby Navajo Sandstone cliffs and domes. Vertical surface fractures aligned at right angles to the cross-bedding (a pattern called checkerboarding) are obvious, but not as well developed as they are along the Zion-Mt. Carmel Highway between the tunnel and the East Entrance of Zion.

From the overlook, return the way you came. ■

Hike 8. Middle Fork Taylor Creek to Double Arch Alcove

Distance	5.6 miles round trip
Elevation gain	720'
Average hiking time	2½ to 3 hours
Difficulty	3
Child rating	3
Best season	April through November
Hazards	Numerous stream crossings

Driving to the trailhead

The Kolob Canyons Road leaves Interstate 15 at exit 40, 19 miles south of Cedar City and 33 miles north of St. George. The Kolob Canyons visitor center, 0.3 mile east of the highway, offers books and maps for sale, backcountry information, and backcountry permits. Visitors must pay the park entrance fee at the visitor center.

Beyond the visitor center, the road quickly ascends into Taylor Creek canyon. After driving 2.3 miles, you reach the spacious trailhead parking area on the left (north) side of the road, indicated by a TAYLOR CREEK TRAIL sign.

Introduction

The trail to Double Arch Alcove is rough but easy to follow, though it involves crossing small Middle Fork Taylor Creek innumerable times. Prime features include two homestead cabins, microclimate areas with vigorous growth of riparian vegetation and conifer forests, a perennial stream, and wildflower-adorned alcoves at the trail's end.

This area is for day use only, and despite its proximity to Interstate 15, the trail generally receives only moderate use, save on holiday weekends.

Description

As at most Zion trailheads, views from this trailhead (5510') are spectacular. To the west, the walls of Taylor Creek canyon frame the bulky, 10,000-foot Pine Valley Mountains; up-canyon to the east the rusty prows of Tucupit and Paria points stand guard over the portals of Taylor Creek's Finger Canyons. Massive Horse Ranch Mountain dominates the northeast skyline, its cliffbound flanks contrasting with the brush-choked dome of its 8740-foot summit, the highest point in Zion. Atop its crest are Zion's youngest sedimentary rocks, sandstones of the Dakota Formation; and younger still are the Quaternary volcanics that crown the summit.

The interior of a deep and shady canyon beckons, and we get underway beyond the trailhead, descending 80 feet into a woodland of Gambel oak, pinyon, and Utah juniper, and soon reaching the banks of Taylor Creek, a small, high-desert stream. As we proceed up the presently broad canyon, we have to hop across the stream time and again. A fine display of seasonal wild-flowers keeps us company, and big sagebrush, greenleaf manzanita, squaw-bush, and Utah serviceberry form an understory of scattered shrubs. The Fremont cottonwoods, those ubiquitous denizens of streams and washes in the Southwest, become increasingly large as we proceed, their deeply fur-rowed boles and excessively branched crowns casting ample shade and form-ing a picturesque foreground to the stark simplicity of soaring canyon walls.

Approaching the confluence of the North and Middle forks of Taylor Creek, we cross back to the north bank and continue eastward, soon passing below the well-preserved structure of Larsen Cabin at 1.25 miles (5620'), a homestead cabin built with white-fir logs in 1929. This cabin and another one upstream are the only evidence of attempted settlement in the Finger Canyons of the Kolob, but these cabins are not the only evidence of man's use of the canyons. Trailside stumps we may have noticed previously attest to a turn-of-the-century logging and sawmill operation in Taylor Creek. Lumber from the canyon helped to build the small town of New Harmony, west of the park at the foot of the Pine Valley Mountains.

From his small cabin, Gustave C. Larsen probably enjoyed the dramat-ic view of Tucupit Point, abruptly rising more than 500 feet above the con-fluence, just as present-day hikers do. Also visible is Horse Ranch Mountain, where an excellent cross-section of five of Zion's nine sedimentary strata is exposed to full view.

Descending slightly from the cabin, we quickly reach Taylor Creek's North Fork. After crossing it, we continue up the Middle Fork on an increas-ingly poor trail. Upstream the canyon becomes much narrower and receives little sunlight. Eventually the trail becomes little more than a boot-beaten path, and we follow it to a bench where we encounter the Arthur Fife cabin at 2.4 miles (5840'), built in 1930 in a thick stand of Douglas-firs. Since the cabin was built on a moist, shady site, it is more deteriorated than the Larsen Cabin. Great salmon-tinted cliffs soar above the cabin, to both the north and the south, and with the onset of autumn, the bushy maples here glow fiery red as well.

Our indistinct path leads quickly from the cabin down to a nearby vig-orous spring issuing from the porous Navajo Sandstone where it interfaces with impermeable Kayenta shales. The stream may be dry above the spring, and we continue to follow the canyon around a prominent southeastward bend, beyond which we leave the canyon floor and quickly climb to the

shady hollow of Double Arch Alcove at 2.8 miles (6050'), a delightful sylvan oasis decorated with white fir and maple.

Beneath the vaulted roof of this deep recess, cliff columbines grow in
profusion, nurtured by moisture seeping and dripping from the alcove's interior. Directly above the alcove lies a shelf upon which Douglas-fir and white
fir grow tall and straight, and above that shelf, a smooth cliff soars skyward
to a large arch perched just below the rim. Evidence of an opening behind
that arch is suggested by a tapestry of streaks left upon the wall below by ages
of mineral-laden runoff that must have flowed through the opening above
the alcove.

From Double Arch Alcove, retrace your steps to the trailhead. ■

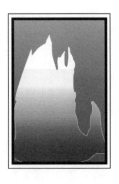

Bryce Canyon
National Park

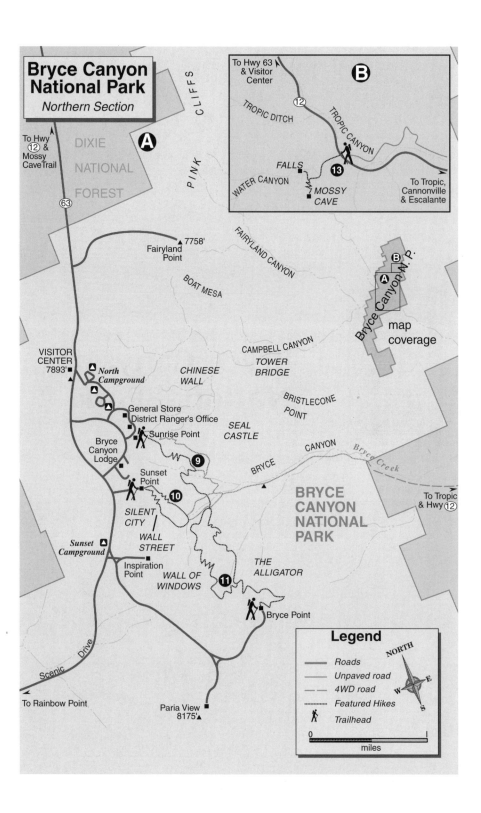

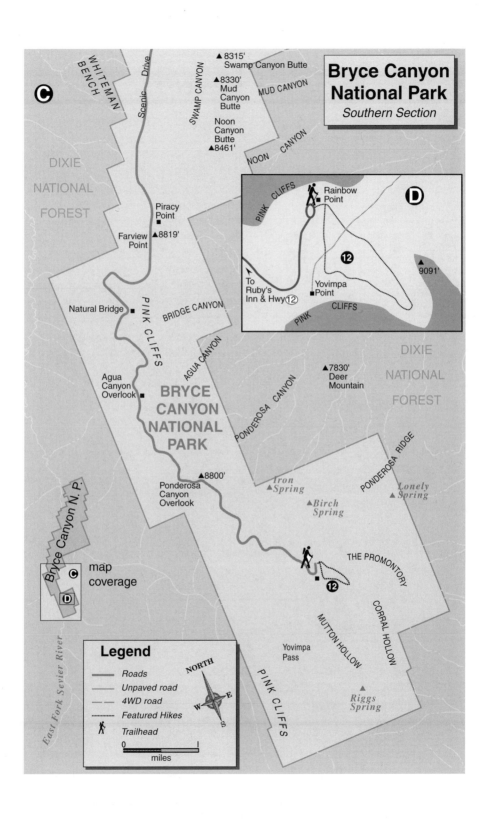

Bryce Canyon
National Park
Southern Section

C

WHITEMAN BENCH

Scenic Drive

SWAMP CANYON

▲ 8315'
Swamp Canyon Butte

▲ 8330'
Mud Canyon Butte

MUD CANYON

Noon Canyon Butte
▲ 8461'

NOON CANYON

DIXIE

NATIONAL

FOREST

Piracy Point

Farview Point ▲ 8819'

PINK CLIFFS

BRIDGE CANYON

Natural Bridge

AGUA CANYON

Agua Canyon Overlook

BRYCE CANYON NATIONAL PARK

PINK CLIFFS

Rainbow Point

D

To Ruby's Inn & Hwy ⑫

⑫

Yovimpa Point

▲ 9091'

PINK CLIFFS

DIXIE

NATIONAL

FOREST

PONDEROSA CANYON

▲ 7830'
Deer Mountain

PONDEROSA RIDGE

▲ 8800'
Ponderosa Canyon Overlook

Iron ▲*Spring*

Lonely ▲ *Spring*

▲*Birch Spring*

Bryce Canyon N. P.

C

map coverage

D

East Fork Sevier River

⑫

THE PROMONTORY

CORRAL HOLLOW

Yovimpa Pass

MUTTON HOLLOW

PINK CLIFFS

▲
Riggs Spring

Legend

— Roads
— Unpaved road
- - - 4WD road
········· Featured Hikes
🚶 Trailhead

NORTH
N
W · E
S

0 _____ 1
miles

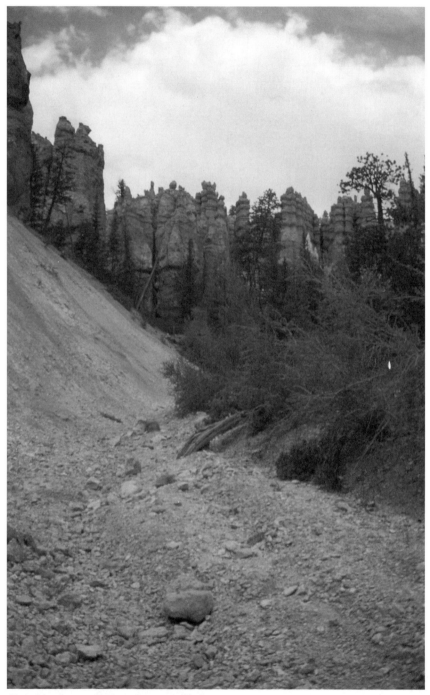

Typical hoodoos in the Bryce Canyon amphitheater

Introduction

Bryce Canyon National Park, located on the east edge of the Paunsaugunt Plateau in south-central Utah, is the smallest of Utah's national parks, with an area of only 35,835 acres (56 square miles). But within the confines of this park is perhaps the most unusual spectacle of erosional forms on earth. Here the optimum combination of rock type and climate has led to the creation of a striking array of pillars, finlike ridges, windows and arches, separated from each other by narrow stone hallways and badlands slopes. These features seem to erupt from the rim of the forested plateau in a colorful, fiery display that at once overwhelms the senses.

Drive to any of the overlooks on the plateau rim and you will be astounded by the profusion of stone pillars at your feet, colored in shades of orange, white, and yellow—colors that assume a wide range of hues with the passing hours of the day. When you have finally recovered from the initial explosion of color and form, other landforms besides Bryce's pillars begin to draw your attention.

Bryce is not only a showcase for and a tribute to nature's unique expression; it is a place where you can revel in a clean environment and absorb far-flung vistas seen through 100 miles of the crystalline air of southern Utah, vistas limited only by the curvature of the earth. Indeed, clean air is a precious resource in our world, and the desert Southwest boasts the cleanest air in the nation.

Unlike Zion and Grand Canyon national parks, Bryce preserves not one canyon but many, all tributaries to the Paria River, which in turn contributes its waters to the mighty Colorado. As these canyons have eroded back into the eastern escarpment of the Paunsaugunt Plateau, they have created a series of basins, exposing naked stone to the elements. Hence, as you drive to the various overlooks on the crenelated rim, you are greeted by a new and unique view in each place.

When you visit Bryce, park your car and walk the trails. Revel in the endless panoramas of the unspoiled Utah landscape; breath deeply of the clean, thin air; watch the shadows of late afternoon creep over the rim and fill the canyon amphitheaters to the brim; immerse yourself in the sounds of the wind rushing among hoodoos and rustling among the pines; gaze in wonder at the gnarled, time-etched bristlecone pines that stand in quiet defiance of the harsh elements; and wander among the sculptured hoodoos that only nature, in her finest erosional sculpturing, could have created.

In a region where thousands of square miles of magnificent red-rock landscapes seem to continually overwhelm the senses, the incomparable Pink Cliffs of Bryce stand out above all the rest, and will draw you back time and again to savor some of nature's secrets.

Plants and animals of Bryce

Bryce's 2500 feet of vertical relief embrace an array of distinctive environments, each one supporting a particular assemblage of vegetation. Woodlands of pinyon, Utah juniper, and Gambel oak occupy the lowest elevations in the park. They dominate the upper limits of the Upper Sonoran life zone, from 6600 to about 7000 feet, where precipitation averages a scant 12 inches, summer temperatures can exceed 100°, and winter temperatures occasionally plunge below 0°. These woodlands thrive on the weathered sandstone that forms a gentle landscape of shallow canyons and broad, rolling ridges well below the breaks of the Pink Cliffs. Few park trails pass through this zone, but the Under-the-Rim Trail frequently touches its fringes.

In the Transition Zone, near the 7000-foot level on the plateau or in the canyons, open, park-like forests of tall ponderosa pines dominate the landscape. An average of more than 15 inches of precipitation nurtures these trees, and due to competition for moisture, they are widely spaced, as are the lower-elevation pinyon and juniper. Rocky Mountain juniper sporadically mixes with ponderosa pines in the Transition zone.

Broad meadows occupy low-lying areas on the plateau in the Transition Zone. The tall, thick grasses of these meadows attracted pioneer stockmen, who grazed their cattle and sheep on the plateau during summer. The present-day sagebrush infestation of the meadows reflects years of overgrazing these grasslands.

Conifers are steadily encroaching upon the sloping margins of the meadows, although the low-lying depressions are generally not conducive to tree growth. These areas are typically wetter than other locations and winter temperature inversions trap cold air and cause it to collect in them. Temperatures can be 30° colder than on surrounding slopes, and the cold can severely retard the establishment of tree seedlings.

In the Canadian Zone, where elevations climb to 9000 feet in the southern reaches of the park, temperatures are cooler still, and precipitation increases markedly from the 15-inch average at the park visitor center. Ponderosa pines are mostly supplanted by conifers that like a cooler, moister environment. The dominant trees in this zone are Douglas-fir and white fir, although ponderosas persist on drier, sun-drenched slopes up to nearly 9000 feet. Aspens occupy this zone's cool, moist draws and meadow margins.

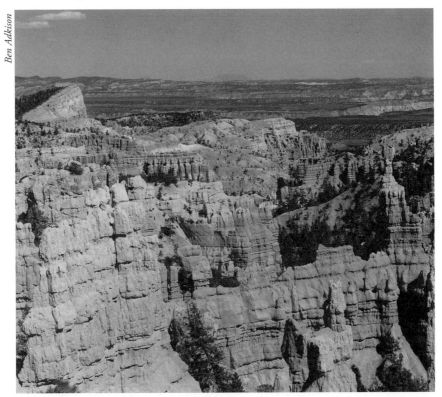

Ben Adkison

Pink cliffs below Sunset Point

The elevation of the Pink Cliffs places them within both the Transition and Canadian life zones, yet the forests of the plateau and the woodlands of the foothills abruptly end in the canyon amphitheaters. The hoodoos and badlands of the Pink Cliffs cannot support forest, and only a few trees and shrubs can survive on this barren land. The tenacious bristlecone and limber pines inhabit the most inhospitable sites on the rim and the breaks of the Pink Cliffs. These trees contend with the harshest environmental conditions anywhere in the park. Remarkably, they thrive on nutrient-poor limestone slopes where most other plants cannot exist.

The bristlecone pine is well adapted to conserve available resources. Needles persist on its branches for 25–30 years, and in drought years the trees add no new growth. When conditions cannot support the growth of an entire tree, it will die back and maintain only enough growth to allow survival; often it seems that only a strip of bark supports a few living branches, while the rest of the tree is merely a wind-polished skeleton of its former self.

Animal life in Bryce is as diverse as its vegetation, and like plant communities, animals have adapted to particular park habitats.

One hundred and seventy species of birds inhabit Bryce National Park. One hundred and eighteen of these species are seasonal visitors; the remaining 52 make Bryce their permanent home. The sudden chortling of the common raven often startles hikers on park trails, and evening visitors to the rim overlooks often see these jet-black birds roosting among the hoodoos below. During fall, the raucous call of pinyon jays filters through the sparse foliage of the pinyon-juniper woodland as they feed on a bounty of pinyon nuts. The mockingbird, Say's phoebe, mountain bluebird, black-capped chickadee, and gray vireo, are less conspicuous denizens of these woodlands, as are the blue grosbeak, house finch, sage sparrow, and rufous-sided towhee. In the meadows, the horned lark, western meadowlark, and sage grouse are joined by mountain bluebird, and loggerhead shrike. The forests are home to the blue grouse, band-tailed pigeon, Williamson's sapsucker, as well as the Steller's jay, gray jay, Clark's nutcracker, brown creeper, and gray junco.

The violet-green swallow and the white-throated swift entertain park visitors near the rim throughout each day during the summer. They perform aerial acrobatics at such incredible speeds that they are usually seen only for a fleeting instant. The white-throated swift can attain speeds of 200 miles per hour while diving for its insect prey.

Forty-nine species of mammals and rodents range on the plateau and traverse the foothills of Bryce. The mule deer is the largest mammal most likely to be seen in Bryce and ranges throughout the park. Diverse shrubs and grasses make the plateau an ideal summer retreat for the deer, and occasionally their chief predator, the mountain lion. During winter, when the plateau is covered in snow, the deer descend into the eastern foothills, where they feed on shrubs such as mountain mahogany and bitterbrush, the seeds of pinyons, and the berries of junipers.

The Rocky Mountain elk is the largest mammal that inhabits the Paunsaugunt Plateau, although it more typically frequents the heights of Sevier Plateau north of Bryce. Pronghorn antelope are also seen, although rarely, on the gentle surface of the Paunsaugunt Plateau. Yellow-bellied marmots and the threatened white-tailed prairie dog make their homes in and around the plateau's grasslands, as do pocket gophers and skunks. Porcupine, spruce squirrels, and northern flying squirrels are specifically adapted to forest environments. Gray fox, long-tailed weasels, golden-mantled ground squirrels, and a variety of chipmunks are also denizens of the plateau's forests. In lower elevations, hikers may encounter coyotes, rock squirrels, desert cottontails, and bobcats.

Bryce boasts 15 species of reptiles and amphibians. The most common reptile seen on the park's trails is the mountain short-horned lizard, an armored reptile that symbolizes the desert to many visitors. The striped whipsnake is a common snake in Bryce. Another, less-welcome sight on the trail is the Great Basin rattlesnake, the only poisonous reptile in the park.

These snakes attain lengths of up to 5½ feet, but their coloration allows them to blend well with their surroundings, and they won't always rattle a warning if one comes too close. Hikers traveling cross-country should be especially careful where they place their hands and feet to avoid an unfortunate encounter with this beautiful but dangerous reptile. Three lizards—side-blotched, northern sagebrush, and northern plateau—are all common in the lower elevations of the park.

All the plants and animals in the park live in a delicate balance, and to disrupt any part of the ecosystem threatens their well-being and consequently, the overall health of the environment. So, while enjoying this unique and exquisite example of nature's handiwork, do all you can not only to preserve it for those who follow, but also to show consideration for the plants and animals that make Bryce their home.

Interpretive activities

A variety of interpretive activities is available in Bryce to enhance your appreciation and knowledge of the dramatic and dynamic processes that have shaped the park in the past, and those that play an important role in the park today.

Every visitor's first stop in Bryce should be at the visitor center. Only 40% of the annual average of nearly one million visitors take advantage of this invaluable facility, where park rangers can answer your questions and help you make the most of your stay. A slide program, interpretive exhibits, and a myriad of publications will help you gain knowledge of every aspect of the park. Schedules of interpretive programs, including guided hikes and evening amphitheater programs, are posted here as well.

The visitor center is open all year, and during the summer season business hours are 8 A.M.–8 P.M. daily. Schedules of interpretive activities are available at the visitor center. Evening talks are conducted nightly at both campground amphitheaters, from May through August or September.

Ranger-led walks offer novice hikers an exceptional opportunity to enjoy Bryce's trails, and allow any hiker to learn more about the park's fascinating geology, flora, and animal and bird populations.

Campgrounds

Bryce's two spacious campgrounds provide 218 campsites, with spaces for RVs and tent camping. A group campsite is available at Sunset Campground. Campers pay the nightly fee at the self-registration station at each campground entrance, but are advised to arrive early in the day as both campgrounds are typically filled by early afternoon during the summer. North Campground, reached via a spur road just south of the visitor center, lies at 7900 feet just west of the plateau rim north of Sunrise Point. It sits in an open forest of ponderosa and limber pines, with a scattering of Rocky Mountain junipers. Short trails lead from the campground to awe-inspiring viewpoints on the Rim Trail. Loop A in the campground remains open all winter. Sunset Campground lies west of the park road, just south of the Sunset Point Road at 8000 feet elevation. It is smaller than North Campground, but it is shaded by a cool forest.

Historic Bryce Canyon Lodge stands at 7978 feet just west of Sunrise Point. Reservations six months or more in advance are recommended for visitors planning to stay at the motel or the western cabins there. The lodge also offers a restaurant, a gift shop, and daily horseback rides on two park trails. Just north of the lodge are a gas station and a general store where showers are available. The lodge usually remains opens from May through mid-October.

A variety of private campgrounds, motels, and restaurants is found along Utah Highway 12 within a few miles of the park. Tropic, Utah, in the valley east of the park, offers several motels, restaurants, groceries, fuel, and vehicle repair and towing.

Ruby's Inn, a short distance north of the park on Utah Highway 63, offers a wide range of services. In addition to a campground, this resort features the amenities of a large town, including two large motels, an RV park; tepees for overnight accommodations, showers, laundry, a general store, a restaurant, two gas stations with diesel fuel and propane available, and towing and repair facilities for cars and RVs. Arrangements can be made there for helicopter rides and rentals of 4-wheel OHVs.

Kings Creek Campground, on East Fork Sevier River in Dixie National Forest, is reached via a 7-mile dirt road that begins 4.5 miles west of the Utah Highways 12/63 junction north of the park. Another Forest Service campground lies alongside Utah 12 in Red Canyon, a few miles east of U.S. 89.

Hiking and backpacking equipment is not available near the park.

For further information, contact:

Park Superintendent
Bryce Canyon National Park
P.O. Box 170001
Bryce Canyon, UT 84717-0001
(435) 834-5322

For information on horseback rides, contact:

Canyon Trail Rides
P.O. Box 128
Tropic, UT 84776-0128
(435) 679-8665

For information on lodging at Bryce Canyon Lodge, contact:
Amfac Parks and Resorts
14001 East Iliff Ave., Suite 600
Aurora, CO 80014-1433
(303) 297-2757
FAX (303) 297-3175

Hiking in Bryce

The park highway offers a variety of scenic overlooks where nonhikers can view the landscape without leaving their cars. But most overlooks require at least a short stroll of 100–200 yards, and most visitors leave their cars for a walk to Sunrise and Sunset points, Inspiration and Bryce points, Paria View, or Rainbow Point.

But these visitors are experiencing Bryce from above; to gain the essential park experience, you must follow the trails into the heart of the breaks, walking among the ranks of pillars, finlike ridges, badlands slopes, and slot canyons. Some visitors, after gazing from the overlooks, come to think that it is all the same, that perhaps the repetition of views is monotonous, and that the canyon amphitheaters offer little more than can be seen from above. But hiking the trails allows an intimate association with the myriad erosional forms and views that change with every bend in the trail.

Bryce's 60 miles of trails offer hiking opportunities ranging from leisurely strolls to backpacks of three or four days. The trail network samples virtually every aspect of park scenery.

Except for the Rim Trail and the Bristlecone Loop Trail, all the park's trails descend from the rim and require a stiff climb to regain it. When you combine the ups and downs with the relative lack of oxygen at the park's high elevations, many of the trails become demanding, even to seasoned hikers.

Some shorter trails into the Bryce Canyon amphitheater are frequently used, including the spectacular Navajo Loop and Queens Garden trails. Somewhat less used trails north of Bryce Point include the longer Peekaboo Loop and Fairyland trails.

South of Bryce Point are the only backpacking trails in the park: Under-the-Rim and Riggs Spring Loop. These trails receive considerably less day-hiking pressure due to their length and their location far below the rim.

Many of the park's shorter trails are wide, smooth, and well-maintained. There are few trails that offer access to wheelchairs. The Rim Trail between Sunrise and Sunset points, 0.5 mile long, is paved, with only minor undulations. Stronger handicapped persons can negotiate the one-mile Bristlecone Loop Trail; however, it has moderate grades, is gravelled, and at one point passes very close to the rim.

Despite the well-watered appearance of the green forests that mantle much of the park, the region is semiarid and the air is dry. When hiking any park trail, always carry adequate water and ample provisions, and wear sturdy shoes or boots.

Bryce is a high-elevation park; summers are generally warm but winters bring deep snow and bitter cold. Average precipitation ranges from 12 inches near the east boundary of the park to nearly 15 inches at the visitor center at 7900 feet, to as much as 25 inches in the high southern reaches of the plateau.

June is the driest month, August the wettest. The summer months of July and August see frequent thunderstorms, when downpours scour the debris from gullies and washes below the rim, and thunder reverberates among the hoodoos. The months of May through August bring more visitors to Bryce than all other months combined, and this summer season is one of the most delightful times to visit the park; days are warm, and the forests and meadows are enriched with colorful flowers.

The sky in the late-summer thunderstorm season displays a dynamic interplay of billowing clouds, sunlight and shadow, lightning, heavy gully-washing rains, and sometimes hail. Thunderstorms typically develop by early afternoon, fed by convection currents of hot air rising from the heated landscape. Since most of the park's trails are exposed and dangerous during thunderstorms, morning hikes are best if thunderstorms are in the forecast.

By autumn, crowds abate, the days are cool, and the oaks, aspens and maples paint the park with colors rivaling those of the Pink Cliffs in brilliance and variety.

Snow typically begins to blanket the landscape by November, and in the winter and early spring months, the park is the realm of cross-country skiers and snowshoers. Popular snow routes in the park include the Fairyland and Paria Point roads and the Rim Trail. The visitor center offers snowshoes on loan to visitors free of charge.

Most park trails are the domain of the hiker, but there are exceptions. The Horse Trail, which descends into Bryce Canyon from Sunrise Point, and the Peekaboo Loop Trail are used twice daily by the park concessioner for trail rides.

There are no toilets on Bryce's backcountry trails. As in all other national parks in Utah, hikers are required to pack out their toilet paper (use zipper-lock plastic bags). ■

Hike 9. Queens Garden Trail

Distance	3.4 miles round trip
Elevation gain	600'
Average hiking time	1½ to 2 hours
Difficulty rating	3
Child rating	2
Best season	May through October
Hazards	Steep dropoffs

Driving to the trailhead

Access to Bryce Canyon National Park is via Utah 63, a paved dead-end road branching south from Utah 12. From the east, that's 47 miles west of Escalante and 7.5 miles west of Tropic. Most park visitors, however, travel from U.S. 89, west of the park. The prominently signed junction of U.S. 89 and Utah 12, in the upper Sevier Valley, lies 44 miles north of Mount Carmel Junction and 61 miles north of Kanab, or 82 miles south of Richfield and 10 miles south of Panguitch. Utah 63 is 14 miles east of U.S. 89 via Utah 12.

From the junction of Utah highways 12 and 63, drive south on Utah 63, passing through the elaborate tourist complex of Ruby's Inn for 2.5 miles to the signed park boundary, where Utah 63 ends and the paved, two-lane park road continues south, climbing gently through a pleasant, open forest of ponderosa pines.

After 2.8 miles the signed road to Fairyland Canyon branches east. Continue past that junction, reaching the park entrance station at 3.6 miles, and passing the visitor center at 3.7 miles. After driving 4.0 miles from Utah 12, turn left onto a signed eastbound spur road leading to the general store and the picnic area. Follow this road for 0.3 mile to a junction with a left-branching road leading to a picnic area and North Campground. Bear right there, and follow the road as it curves south toward Bryce Canyon Lodge. After another 0.25 mile turn left, curving upward (north) toward the District Ranger's Office (DRO) and the general store. Opposite the DRO, after a final 0.2 mile, you reach a large parking area just below Sunrise Point.

Introduction

This is a popular dayhike into the incomparable Bryce Canyon amphitheater, descending into the realm of hoodoos, castles, and balanced rocks, many of which have been likened to familiar images and given such fanciful names as Gullivers Castle and Queen Victoria.

Many hikers combine the Queens Garden Trail with a leg of the Navajo Loop Trail (Hike 10) and loop back to Sunrise Point via the Rim Trail. Others, if they don't mind meeting horses and hiking a dusty trail, can loop back to the trailhead via the mile-long Horse Trail, a route that few hikers tread. The minor inconvenience of possibly encountering horseback riders from the lodge is more than compensated for by striking landscapes and exceptional views. Whichever route hikers choose, they will be rewarded by some of the most awe-inspiring scenery the park has to offer.

Description

From the parking area just southeast of the general store and the District Ranger's Office (7950'), hike past a SUNRISE POINT sign. Follow the paved trail southeast for 150 yards to a fork and bear right, quickly reaching the Rim Trail. (The left fork also leads to the Rim Trail.) Immediately beyond this junction, a trail forks right toward Bryce Lodge, and the Horse Trail quickly forks left, descending from the rim. Ignoring both trails, proceed south along the rim. Climb gently to a junction with the Queens Garden Connecting Trail at 0.2 mile (8000'), immediately before reaching Sunrise Point. Turning right on that trail, we descend moderately along or near a ridge that plunges eastward from Sunrise Point. We will enjoy ever-changing views as we proceed, including Queens Garden, Bryce Point, and the forested floor of Bryce Canyon to the south. The colorful Campbell Canyon drainage and Boat Mesa lie to the northeast, and distant panoramas include the Table Cliffs, Canaan Peak, and Tropic Valley.

After descending a series of switchbacks, we traverse badlands slopes decorated by ponderosa and bristlecone pines beneath isolated hoodoos, soon passing directly below towering Gullivers Castle and a notch in the ridge framing orange, fluted cliffs westward below the tree-studded rim, then reach the signed junction at 0.8 mile (7680') with the trail to Queens Garden.

Turn right at the junction and descend to the realm of Queens Garden via a series of short switchbacks, which soon lead through a short tunnel. The trail winds downward among the recesses of the garden, where a myriad of starkly beautiful castles, towers, pillars, minarets, and fins, colored in shades of orange and white, stir the imagination. Dark-green conifers contrast with these colorful erosional forms, growing vigorously in intervening gullies and sparsely on nearby slopes.

Bending into a south-trending draw, we traverse southward around the nose of a ridge and pass through another tunnel before bending northwest back into another draw. Many hoodoos in the park are "primary wall-type" hoodoos—narrow, finlike ridges projecting outward from the rim. Here there is a concentration of pinnacles, towers, castles, and spires, and their walls are irregularly fluted. Colors range from shades of white to yellow and orange. Queens Garden is composed generally of the eroded remnants of such finlike ridges, eroded to the point that the hoodoos are largely isolated from one another by intervening badlands slopes and saddles.

Curving southward out of this draw, we pass through a third tunnel and quickly reach a junction at 1.2 miles (7600'). A spur trail forks right here, signed for Queen Victoria, while the main trail is signed for the Navajo Loop Trail. This spur leads northwest up a small draw, dead-ending after 100 yards beneath the namesake of this northernmost lobe of the Bryce amphitheater, Queen Victoria. Bearing a striking resemblance to the 19th century monarch, the "Queen," wearing a crown of whitish stone, watches over her realm from atop the northernmost of four prominent pinnacles rising immediately east of the trail's end.

Returning to the main trail, continue southward, bound for the Navajo Loop Trail, at first descending gently along a dry gully. The trail briefly narrows where two orange hoodoos close in, then continues downhill amid tall conifers and taller hoodoos.

After we stroll south for a few minutes from the Queen Victoria spur trail, a sign carved into a trailside stump points the way to the Navajo Loop Trail. Soon thereafter a sign indicating the Horse Trail marks a junction with a spur trail forking left into Bryce Canyon at 1.6 miles (7400'). Hikers now have the choice of (1) turning left onto the aforementioned spur trail to reach the Horse Trail, which loops back to the trailhead in 1.4 very scenic miles; or (2) retracing their steps back to the trailhead. ■

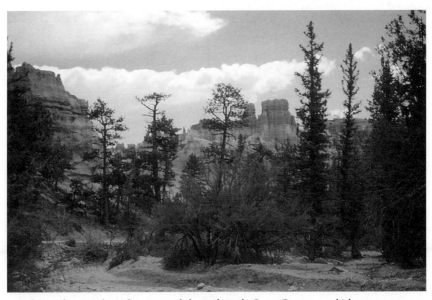

Hoodoos and scattered conifers surround the trails in the Bryce Canyon amphitheater

Hike 10. Navajo Loop Trail

Distance	1.5 miles loop trip
Elevation gain	550'
Average hiking time	1 to 1½ hours
Difficulty rating	3
Child rating	2
Best season	May through October
Hazards	Steep dropoffs

Driving to the trailhead

Follow driving directions for Hike 9 to reach Utah Highway 63 leading to Bryce Canyon National Park. Follow Utah 63 and the paved park road south from Utah 12 for 4.8 miles to an eastbound spur road signed for Sunset Point. Leave the park road there, turn left, and drive 0.2 mile to the large parking area at the roadend loop, from where three improved trails quickly lead to Sunset Point and the Rim Trail.

Introduction

This popular, short dayhike offers ample rewards for a modicum of effort. Passing the crumbling stone edifices of Silent City, the shadow-filled hallway of Wall Street, the water-carved spans of Two Bridges, and the balanced rock of Thors Hammer (to name but a few of the remarkable erosional features passed enroute) this trip packs more exceptional scenery into a short hike than perhaps any other trail in the park.

Description

From the large parking area at the end of the Sunset Point spur road (7995') three paved trails lead east for 125 yards to the rim at Sunset Point, where they meet the Rim Trail going left and right.

Just north of the extensive fenced-in viewing area of Sunset Point, the signed, wide, and well-maintained Navajo Loop Trail departs downhill, switchbacking down the first cliff band below the rim, its moist and sheltered microclimate harboring stunted aspens at its base. After about 125 yards, the trail forks. The left fork continues descending, while the right fork quickly traverses toward a U-shaped gap between colorful hoodoos. Wall Street and the Silent City beckon, so for now we'll take the right fork.

Passing through a hoodoo-rimmed notch, we stand above the maze of Silent City, where dark, narrow defiles separate finlike cliffs that are as high as 200 feet. At the notch another wide trail forks right, quickly ending in the tunnel visible ahead. Seen from the tunnel, a myriad of tall, fanciful pinnacles rise out of Silent City, their summits just below eye level. This bewildering semicircular array of pinnacles is laced with many deep, dark, mysterious chasms, their shady depths virtually unknown.

The Navajo Loop Trail then descends a steep, orange-colored slope via 29 short, tight switchbacks. Pinnacles tower higher above as we descend past huge boulders. We go down this well-designed series of switchbacks into the heart of Silent City, flanked by colorful limestone cliffs.

Below the switchbacks, the trail enters the dark, narrow passage of Wall Street. The cliffs in Wall Street, as in the rest of Bryce, are not smooth but have wrinkled, corrugated surfaces. Here tall cliffs rise steeply over 100 feet above and stand barely 20 feet apart. Some hikers may feel claustrophobic in this chasm, but its cool, shady depths are attractive on a hot summer day. Here we gain a close-up look at the varicolored layers of the Claron Formation, sediments laid down at the bottom of ancient lakes and streams between about 60 and 40 million years ago.

The bottom of Wall Street has been scoured over the years by floodwaters, and as a result the cliffs above overhang our trail in places. As we proceed into Wall Street we'll pass a few tall, vigorous Douglas-firs, their straight trunks free of branches, their crowns reaching for sunlight near the top of the fluted cliffs.

Leaving the confines of Wall Street, we turn southeast to join a larger wash draining the rim. Compared to Wall Street, this wash enjoys considerable sunlight, which encourages a diverse forest here, aided by deeper sediments in which trees can gain a foothold and by a concentration of moisture at the foot of cliffs. The dark-green foliage of Douglas-fir, ponderosa and limber pine, juniper and a few spruces frame the colorful pinnacles rising above us. Manzanita carpets the orange-tinted ground, and scattered boulders fallen from the cliffs above attest to the inexorable forces that are constantly reshaping the landscape.

Ahead our trail rounds the abrupt terminus of a southeast-trending ridge and we stroll northeast to a four-way junction at 0.8 mile (7475'). Following the signed Navajo Loop Trail past the junction, we climb to the left (northwest) into a tree-shaded canyon bounded by a fascinating array of erosional forms. Soon it appears we are heading into a box canyon with no way out, but the trail finds a narrow passageway among colorful minarets. After we enter this narrow defile, numerous gullies feed the main drainage.

A sign points to Two Bridges, a short distance up one of these side gullies (0.2 mile from the junction). A quick stroll up this gorge reveals the bridges, which are composed of one of the more resistant layers of the Claron Formation. Drainage in the gully has worn away a softer layer under-

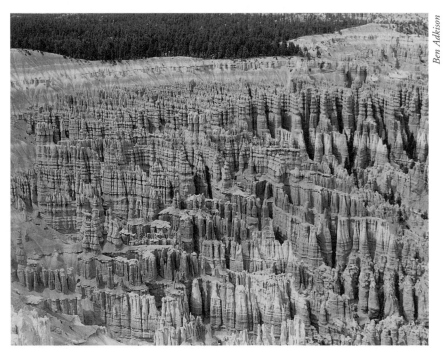

Ben Adkison

Silent City from Inspiration Point, Rim Trail

neath. The span of the larger bridge is about 20 feet high, while that of the smaller bridge is only 4 feet above the floor of the gully.

Above Two Bridges, the Navajo Loop Trail climbs moderately steeply up a gully reminiscent of Wall Street. A series of short switchbacks ensue, and hikers pausing to catch their breath may notice Oregon grape thriving in shady nooks along the way. At the top of this stiff climb, we traverse beneath castle-like hoodoos and notice an especially striking finger-like pinnacle rising above the trail—The Sentinel. We then pass a few windows and gaze northward to prominent Thors Hammer, beyond which stands The Pope, clad in a white "robe," and dozens of other startlingly familiar erosional forms. One final switchback leads us to the junction below Sunset Point, where we bear right to retrace our route to the Sunset Point parking area at 1.5 miles. ■

Hike 11. Peekaboo Loop Trail

Distance	5.0 miles semiloop trip
Elevation gain	850'
Average hiking time	2½ to 3 hours
Difficulty rating	4
Child rating	3
Best season	May through October
Hazards	Steep dropoffs

Driving to the trailhead

Follow driving directions for Hike 9 to reach Utah Highway 63 leading to Bryce Canyon National Park. Follow Utah 63 and the paved park road south from Utah 12 for 5.3 miles to the signed junction with a left-branching spur road leading to Inspiration Point, Bryce Point, and Paria View.

Turn left here, and almost at once reach a junction with the Inspiration Point spur road, which ends in a loop just below the plateau rim after 0.3 mile, offering access to the Rim Trail. Bearing right at that junction, the road ascends gently, soon skirting the foot of badlands slopes.

After driving 1.3 miles from the main park road you reach roads forking right to Paria View and left to Bryce Point. Bearing left onto the Bryce Point Road, you climb for 0.6 mile to the large trailhead parking area just below Bryce Point.

Introduction

This superb dayhike tours the southern half of Bryce Canyon amphitheater. It passes numerous springs, traverses shady microclimates that host Colorado blue spruce and white fir, winds among a colorful collection of hoodoos, and crosses badlands slopes.

Just before climbing back to the rim, hikers find a picnic table and a drinking fountain in a draw below a perennial spring, a fine place for a rest before the stiff climb. Don't rely on the drinking fountain for water; bring your own water.

Description

To reach the Peekaboo Loop Trail, we depart from the east side of the Bryce Point parking area (8300'), and follow a dirt trail, heading steadily downhill via steps toward the southeast. At a signed junction at 0.1 mile

(8235'), we part ways with the Under-the-Rim Trail and bear left onto the Peekaboo Connecting Trail.

Beyond the junction, the wide, smooth, dirt-surface trail leads through an open forest of ponderosa, limber, and bristlecone pines and Douglas-fir. A series of switchbacks soon follows, and they serve to lower us over the rim where white dolomitic slopes give way to the more colorful, iron-rich strata of the Claron Formation.

Soon we descend north-facing slopes via two long switchbacks, and the vegetation begins to reflect a cool and sheltered microclimate. We shortly begin a protracted traverse high above a forested, hoodoo-rimmed canyon. Enroute we pass through a short tunnel bored through a knife-edged ridge, where a resistant orange layer and a crumbly lavender layer of the Claron Formation coalesce. Beyond the tunnel, our gaze stretches into the forested canyons below, including the aptly named Alligator, a white dolomite-capped hoodoo.

The trail leads across the mud and runoff from an upslope spring, and enroute we briefly spy the fenced overlook of Bryce Point, now 400 feet above, atop steep white cliffs. Trees are scattered on these steep slopes, and the few shrubs that are able to grow here include bitterbrush and mountain spray, the latter with dense, fragrant clusters of small white flowers during summer.

Adding to the dramatic overviews of the hoodoo-filled amphitheater, a variety of summer wildflowers will delight our senses as well, including tall, red Wyoming paintbrush, and the yellow blooms of groundsel, hymenopappus, and gumweed.

Soon the trail curves southwest around a steep ridge that plunges below Bryce Point. Gazing beyond the steep draw that lies before us, we see two prominent white pillars below the rim. Between them is one of many arches and windows that penetrate the finlike ridges of Bryce. A keyhole-shaped window lies just south of the above-mentioned window, and numerous alcoves incise the cliffs under the rim. Soon the Wall of Windows comes into view, where two openings frame the sky beyond.

Switchbacks ensue amid colorful hoodoos crowned by resistant caprocks, and we soon reach a junction at 1.0 mile (7680') with the loop trail. Taking the right fork, we descend via switchbacks amid multihued hoodoos. Many hoodoos in Bryce have been given imaginative names, and as we proceed through this wondrous landscape, our imagination likens these landforms to recognizable people and familiar features such as castles and temples.

Highlighting the intervening slopes and gullies between the hoodoos are stands of Douglas-fir, limber and ponderosa pines, and Colorado blue spruce. We soon reach the comparatively level ground of the Bryce Canyon floor in a forest of mixed conifers. Ponderosa pine comes to dominate the forest as we descend into a warmer and drier environment, and 0.4 mile from the junction we cross the canyon's wash, seasonally dampened by the runoff from an upstream spring. But we soon leave the wash, traversing northwest into another draw, where the wide trail, dusty from daily horse traffic, climbs a south-facing slope beneath striking hoodoos. The harsh environment of nearby slopes permits little vegetation other than widely scattered shrubs and stunted trees.

After contouring into another draw, the trail ascends northward. During the climb we'll have fine views south beyond eye-level hoodoos into the colorful recesses of the Bryce amphitheater. A few switchbacks ensue, leading us to a short tunnel and subsequently to a hoodoo-decorated traverse, ending on a ridge just west of the orange tower of Fairy Castle. Views from this ridge extend from Boat Mesa in the north, past Sunrise and Sunset points, to Bryce Point in the south—an engaging panorama encompassing one of the finest erosional spectacles to be seen on the globe.

Descending colorful slopes via switchbacks, we reach a forested draw and drop to a signed junction at 2.3 miles (7440'). From here a short spur leads north less than 100 yards to another junction. The left fork at this junction joins the Navajo Loop Trail, 0.25 mile west. The right fork leads northeast down Bryce Canyon 0.1 mile to a northbound horse trail, then another 0.1 mile to a northwest-bound horse trail, and another 1.2 miles east to a roadend west of Tropic.

We turn left (west) on the return leg of our loop tour, moderately ascending northwest-facing slopes under a shady canopy of ponderosa pines. After 0.3 mile we climb two switchbacks, gaining a northwest view of the Navajo Loop Trail. We can trace its course from Bryce Canyon to Wall Street, where it disappears in the shady recesses of Silent City. The hoodoos and narrow defiles of Silent City rise in a colorful procession of orange, gray, white, and yellow rocks toward serrated ranks of fins jutting outward from the forested rim. A pause here also reveals the butte of Boat Mesa to the north beyond the colorful ridge north of Bryce Canyon.

Continuing our journey, we glimpse Inspiration Point's overlook perched on the rim above to the west, and proceed southward beneath a row of striking orange hoodoos, dominated by The Cathedral. Soon we gain the crest of a north-trending ridge and continue deeper into the mysterious realm of multihued, upright rock formations. Ponderosa and limber pines, Douglas-firs, and blue spruces are scattered but still offer occasional respite from the penetrating Utah sun.

Pause to view the prominent, very steep gully plunging from the rim west of Bryce Point. Here the Peekaboo Fault has slightly offset the strata, and the fault is most easily observed in the offset cliff bands below the steep white slopes abutting the rim. Our trail ahead gently rises and falls, passes through a tunnel in a ridge below Wall of Windows and switchbacks down a narrow, spruce-clad gully. A spire-topped window juts outward from the rim to the south, while Bryce Point rises 700 feet above on the southeast skyline. At the foot of this gully, we turn west and steadily ascend another draw beneath Wall of Windows, thrusting its sheer, fluted cliffs to the sky.

Soon we top out between trailside hoodoos, then traverse 600 feet below the rim, splashing through the runoff of a spring enroute. Bending northeast, our traverse terminates as we descend a sparsely wooded draw and reach a signed junction at 3.9 miles (7600') just above a corral and a pipe-fed water trough. Here we can turn right and follow the spur trail south for 150 yards to a fine rest spot, featuring two picnic tables, toilets, and a spring-fed drinking fountain, shaded by conifers. The trickle of an upstream spring and the breezes through the trees make this a particularly peaceful locale, seemingly a world apart from the hustle and bustle of visitors at Bryce Point, visible nearly 700 feet above.

Returning to the main trail, we skirt the corral, pass a sign pointing to the rim, and quickly hop across a mossy seep from the spring above. We climb gently through the forest and soon reach the terminus of the loop at 4.0 miles (7680'). From there we backtrack the 1-mile view-filled ascent to Bryce Point. ■

Hike 12. Bristlecone Loop Trail

Distance	1.0 mile loop trip
Elevation gain	115'
Average hiking time	30 to 40 minutes
Difficulty rating	2
Child rating	1 to 2
Best season	May through October
Hazards	Steep dropoffs; rim prone to lightning strikes

Driving to the trailhead

Follow driving directions for Hike 9 to reach Utah Highway 63 leading to Bryce Canyon National Park. Follow Utah 63 and the paved park road south from Utah 12 for 19.9 miles to Rainbow Point parking area at the south end of the park road.

Introduction

Bristlecone pines are among the oldest and most enduring living things on earth. Specimens in the Great Basin mountain ranges of California and Nevada have clung to life for nearly 5000 years, but in Bryce the oldest known bristlecone is "only" about 1700 years old, a mere youngster. This enjoyable and easy stroll not only passes among ancient, gnarled bristlecone pines but traverses cool fir forests as well. The trail differs from most park trails in that it traverses the rim rather than descending into the Pink Cliffs below. This trail is also the highest-elevation path in the park, remaining above 9000 feet throughout. In addition, the route offers unique vistas of the southern reaches of the park and the rugged Pink Cliffs, aerial-like vistas of the mesas and cliffs of the Grand Staircase, and a different and more intimate perspective of the Rainbow and Yovimpa Point high country than the often-crowded overlook at Rainbow Point provides.

Description

At the northeast corner of the Rainbow Point parking area and just north of the picnic area (9115'), the Under-the-Rim, Riggs Spring Loop, and Bristlecone Loop trails begin at the destination and mileage sign.

The trail leads through the shady forest for 100 yards to a junction where a sign points right to Yovimpa Point and left to the Under-the-Rim Trail. We will be returning via the right fork, but for now we continue along the left branch, briefly skirting the plateau rim. Views enroute extend northwest to the lofty 11,000- and 12,000-foot summits of the Tushar Mountains, far across the broad forested expanse of the Paunsaugunt Plateau. The trail here is smooth and rock-lined as it descends gently beneath a canopy of Douglas-fir and white fir.

After 200 yards, we part company with hikers on the Under- the-Rim Trail and continue straight ahead on the central trail, signed BRISTLECONE LOOP. The trail branching sharply to our right (southwest) is a cutoff trail leading 350 yards to scenic Yovimpa Point.

Our trail leads us quickly into a shallow draw, then to a gently descending traverse around the shoulder of a minor ridge. We reach a fenced overlook at 0.4 mile (9000'), perched on the rim and featuring a shelter with log benches. The dramatic vista that presently unfolds reaches into the tree-clad depths of Corral Hollow 1000 feet below, seen beyond plunging white cliffs, boulder-strewn orange slopes, and finally ranks of salmon-tinted pillars standing silent guard over Corral Hollow like so many sentinels gazing across distant, undefiled panoramas.

The trail ahead climbs gently to another overlook with far-ranging panoramas framed by sun-burnished snags. Tenacious limber and bristlecone pines also cling stubbornly to existence on this high, weather-tortured promontory. Both trees have needles in bundles of five, but the bristlecone needles are dark green and tufted at the tips of the branches, resembling a fox's tail. The bristlecones are also quite spindly, and some survive only by virtue of a single strip of trunk bark nurturing a few slow-growing branches.

Presently the trail curves northwest, soon passing north of the small air-quality building, where a camera monitors visibility throughout the day. The desert Southwest boasts the best visibility in the nation, attested to by our view of Navajo Mountain over 80 miles distant. Bryce lies within a federally designated Class I air-quality area, and thus is "protected" from degradation of air quality. However, some areas within our view are allowed minimal degradation of air quality, and emissions from distant coal-fired power plants occasionally obscure distant vistas from the park. Grand Staircase-Escalante National Monument encompasses much of our view from east to south. The monument contains vast reserves of gas, oil, and coal, but guidelines restrict the development of those resources, protecting future degradation of the pristine landscapes and clean air we presently enjoy.

Passing a few trailside spruces, we soon leave the rim and re-enter forest, and shortly thereafter reach another four-way junction at 0.8 mile (9090'). The right-branching, previously mentioned cutoff trail leads back to the lower segment of our loop in less than 0.1 mile. The left fork leads 50 yards southwest to the Yovimpa Point Trail. To conclude the loop, however, we follow the center fork through shady forest, soon reaching the trailhead and parking area after 1.0 mile. ■

Hike 13. Water Canyon, Mossy Cave

Distance	1.0 mile round trip to cave and water-fall
Elevation gain	150′
Average hiking time	30 to 40 minutes
Difficulty rating	1
Child rating	1 to 2
Best season	Mid-April through October
Hazards	Steep dropoffs; no water

Driving to the trailhead

Follow driving directions for Hike 9 to reach the Utah Highway 12/63 junction north of Bryce Canyon National Park. Proceed east on Utah 12 from its junction with Utah 63, heading across the open, shrub-clad plateau. In less than a mile, the highway enters Bryce Canyon National Park, and shortly thereafter you breach the Pink Cliffs and begin a steady descent into Tropic Canyon.

Soon the road follows the broad, dry wash of Tropic Canyon, and 3.7 miles from Utah 63, a small sign indicating Mossy Cave directs you to the trailhead parking area, lying on the west side of the road just south of the Water Canyon bridge.

Introduction

Before 1892 Water Canyon was just another dry canyon lying in the rainshadow of the Paunsaugunt Plateau. But farmers in the Paria Valley needed more water for their thirsty fields than the few streams in the valley could provide, so a few valley settlers diverted the waters of East Fork Sevier River into Water Canyon via the Tropic Ditch. Today the canyon boasts a vigorous stream thanks to the ditch, and its waterfalls and cascades are a delight to hikers treading this short but scenic trail. The canyon has its share of salmon-tinted hoodoos, and a scattering of pine woodlands as well.

Mossy Cave is one of the highlights of the canyon, where a continuous supply of dripping water in a deep, cool alcove supports lush, water-loving vegetation seemingly out of place in a high desert environment.

In the past, flash floods have washed away parts of the trail and the two foot bridges spanning Water Canyon's stream. If you visit following a major flood, expect the trail to be more demanding, with the possibility of fording the stream, until Park Service trail crews can reconstruct the trail.

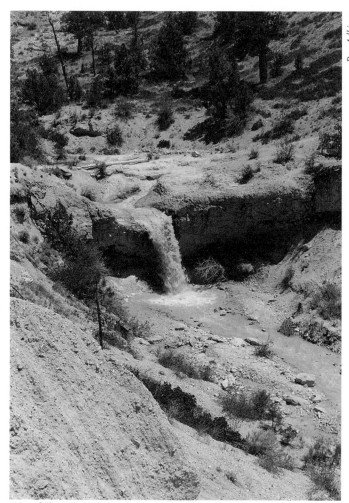

Ben Adkison

Waterfall in Water Canyon

Description

Beginning at the mouth of Water Canyon (6823'), the trail proceeds west through a sunny opening. Picturesque hoodoos in shades of orange and white highlight the slopes of a ridge that rises 300 feet north of the canyon, while to our south, a few limber and bristlecone pines grow on the steep badlands slopes. Small water-loving trees, such as water birch and willows, have found the moist banks of this man-made stream to be an ideal habitat.

Within 200 yards we cross the stream via a sturdy wooden bridge. From here we can see three small windows piercing a prominent salmon-hued hoodoo upslope to our west. The falls in the canyon lie on the opposite side (west) of that hoodoo, and we'll soon be there.

After 0.3 mile we bridge the creek for a second time, pausing to admire the upstream waterfall. After crossing the bridge, we notice false Solomon's seal enjoying the moist, shady environment along the trail.

A brief climb above the bridge brings us to a signed junction: left to Mossy Cave and right to the waterfall. Turning left, we ascend northwest-facing slopes densely clad in juniper, Gambel oak, and ponderosa pine, climbing steeply before we round a bend and are confronted by the dark, dripping alcove of Mossy Cave. A short traverse leads us to the trail's end in the "cave" at 0.4 mile.

This cool, verdant oasis is a delight on the hottest summer days. Here an orange cliff has been hollowed out to make a deep alcove by seeping water that has dissolved the cementing agents that bound the ancient lakebed sediments into stone. Constantly dripping water supports a thick coating of moss in the shady alcove, and we may see the delicate bog orchid thriving in the damp soil nearby. A thick stand of water birch shades the shallow canyon below the cave, while tall ponderosa pines and Douglas-firs grow from the canyon floor to meet the sun above the rim of the cave.

Few hikers bypass the waterfall a short distance up Water Canyon, a delightful rarity in this semiarid land. To get there, head upstream (left, north) from the junction, splashing through the runoff of an upslope spring and reaching the 10-foot waterfall after 0.1 mile, at the point where the stream bends from south to west. Here the blustering creek is backdropped by a scenic cluster of hoodoos rising to the east and pierced by three small windows. The main trail ends just above the waterfall, but a use trail continues upstream, passing among multihued hoodoos on sparsely forested slopes.

This canyon receives little precipitation and is relatively dry, due to its low elevation and location east of the Paunsaugunt Plateau; the scattered forest reflects the competition for this precious moisture. Strong hikers can follow Water Canyon all the way to the rim, but it is quite steep and narrow in its upper reaches, and the rocks of the Claron Formation are often crumbly. A number of side canyons offer interesting explorations.

The upper canyon gives hikers a feeling of discovery that is rare in a heavily trailed national park such as Bryce; since most park visitors aren't even aware of the canyon, and those who are rarely travel beyond Mossy Cave or the falls, hikers who venture into the upper reaches of the canyon will likely enjoy solitude—a precious commodity in the park. ∎

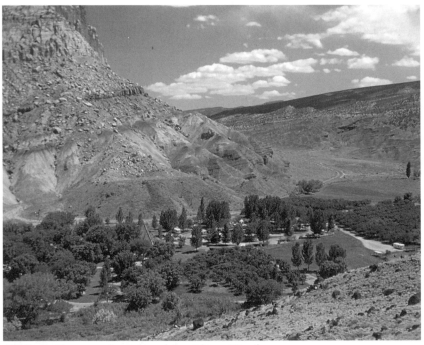

The Fruita Campground spreads out below Johnson Mesa from the Fremont Gorge Viewpoint Trail

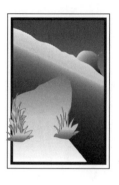

Capitol Reef
National Park

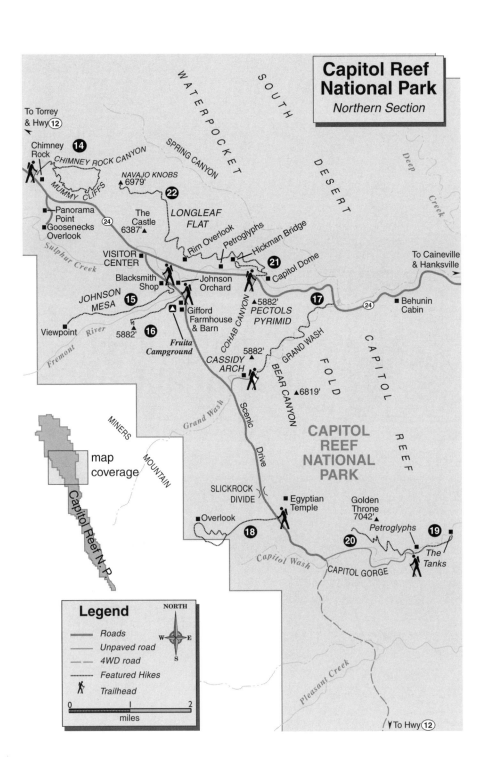

Capitol Reef National Park
Northern Section

To Torrey & Hwy (12)

WATERPOCKET

SOUTH DESERT

Deep Creek

Chimney Rock **14**

CHIMNEY ROCK CANYON

MUMMY CLIFFS

SPRING CANYON

NAVAJO KNOBS ▲6979'

22

LONGLEAF FLAT

Panorama Point
Goosenecks Overlook

(24)

The Castle 6387'▲

Rim Overlook
Petroglyphs
Hickman Bridge

Capitol Dome

To Caineville & Hanksville

Sulphur Creek

VISITOR CENTER

Blacksmith Shop

Johnson Orchard

21

17

(24)

Behunin Cabin

JOHNSON MESA **15**

Gifford Farmhouse & Barn

COHAB CANYON

▲5882' PECTOLS PYRIMID

GRAND WASH

CAPITOL REEF

Viewpoint

Fremont River

5882'▲ **16**

Fruita Campground

CASSIDY ARCH

5882'▲

BEAR CANYON

▲6819'

FOLD

MINERS MOUNTAIN

Grand Wash

Scenic Drive

CAPITOL REEF NATIONAL PARK

map coverage

Capitol Reef N.P.

SLICKROCK DIVIDE

Egyptian Temple

Golden Throne 7042'▲

Petroglyphs **19**

Overlook

18

20

The Tanks

Capitol Wash

CAPITOL GORGE

Pleasant Creek

To Hwy (12)

Legend

NORTH

W E
S

—— Roads
—— Unpaved road
- - - 4WD road
.... Featured Hikes
🚶 Trailhead

0   1   2
miles

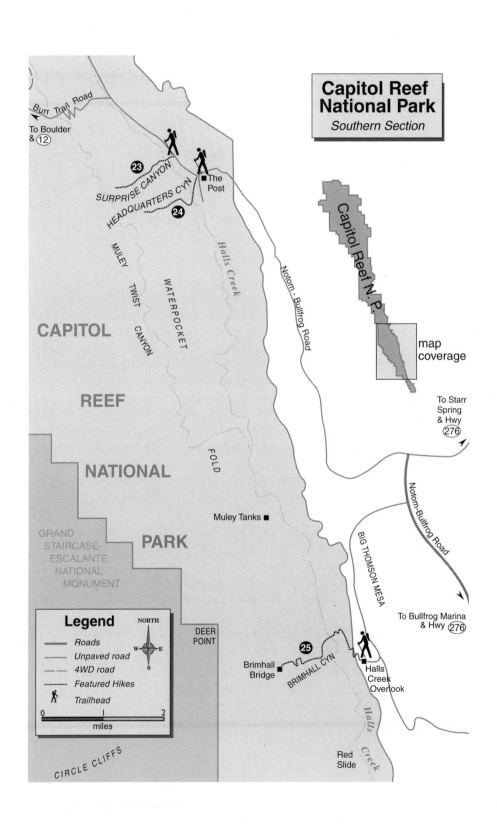

Capitol Reef National Park
Southern Section

Burr Trail Road

To Boulder & (12)

(23)

SURPRISE CANYON

HEADQUARTERS CYN

(24)

■ The Post

Capitol Reef N.P.

map coverage

Halls Creek

MULEY

TWIST

CANYON

WATERPOCKET

CAPITOL

REEF

Notom - Bullfrog Road

To Starr Spring & Hwy (276)

NATIONAL

FOLD

Notom-Bullfrog Road

PARK

GRAND STAIRCASE-ESCALANTE NATIONAL MONUMENT

Muley Tanks ■

BIG THOMSON MESA

To Bullfrog Marina & Hwy (276)

Legend

NORTH

— Roads
— Unpaved road
- - 4WD road
······ Featured Hikes
🚶 Trailhead

W—E
S

DEER POINT

(25)

Brimhall Bridge ■

BRIMHALL CYN

🚶

■ Halls Creek Overlook

0   1   2
miles

CIRCLE CLIFFS

Halls Creek

Red Slide

Introduction

While many Colorado Plateau national parks contain prominent canyons that have been incised deeply into the generally flat landscape, Capitol Reef's 241,671 acres encompass the bulk of the Waterpocket Fold, a 100-mile-long crest of slickrock that resembles a low but incredibly rugged mountain range.

The Waterpocket Fold is an immense bulge in the earth's crust—a monocline—in which 14 sedimentary strata were tilted upward toward the west. Three types of crustal folds are common throughout the Colorado Plateau: in an anticline, the rock layers are buckled upward, forming an elevated ridge; in a syncline, the strata are warped downward, forming a valley or depression; and in a monocline, the strata are tilted upward and then level off at a higher elevation, rather than slanting up or down on both sides. The Capitol Reef landscape, with its sheer slickrock cliffs, towering domes, and blind canyons, was a major barrier to early east-west travel in the region. Hence the name "reef," a term applied to many such natural obstacles on the Colorado Plateau.

The park embraces not only the slickrock spine of the Waterpocket Fold and innumerable slot canyons, but also the extensive desert valleys of South Desert and Strike Valley east of the fold, and the incomparable Cathedral Valleys, where great red monoliths jut skyward from the desert floor like teeth.

South of the Fremont River, the fold narrows considerably as it winds southeastward toward the Colorado River. East of the fold in this area are several other "reefs" that wind through the desert valley that the fold bounds, and each consists of erosional remnants of younger strata that were folded in conjunction with the Waterpocket Fold monocline. East of these minor folds, the landscape abruptly assumes the more uniform character typical of the Colorado Plateau: still younger strata form broad, cliff-edged mesas that rise steadily one after another toward the lofty Henry Mountains.

Visitors who travel off the beaten track to this isolated park will be richly rewarded, not only by some of the grandest scenery on the globe, but perhaps also by introspection and self-discovery that can be achieved only in a land as empty, still, and majestic as Capitol Reef.

Capitol Reef is a not only a celebration of the unique geologic forces that have shaped the land, but also a land that is alive with hardy desert dwellers, both plant and animal, and a region rich in history, stretching back more than 1000 years.

Plants and animals of Capitol Reef

Capitol Reef is home to at least 800 species of plants, which is remarkable considering the park's dry climate; an average of only 7 inches of moisture falls annually at the visitor center. Throughout the park, however, there is a variety of landscapes and soil types (derived from 14 different sedimentary rock layers) and a range of habitats, from perennial streams to deep, shady canyons, badlands slopes, slickrock domes, mesas, and grassy desert valleys.

The Transition and Canadian life zones predominate at the park's highest elevations, on the eastern slopes of 11,306-foot Thousand Lake Mountain. The few hikers who explore these heights will find ancient bristlecone pines—twisted and weather-tortured—and stands of Douglas-fir, Rocky Mountain maple, ponderosa pine, aspen, and Rocky Mountain juniper. (See "Plants and Animals of Zion" above for more on life zones.) The Upper Sonoran Zone encompasses most of the park, dominated by pinyon-juniper woodlands, shrubs, and grass communities.

In all life zones, narrow canyons, stream courses, springs and seeps in this parched desert region support a variety of plants that have one thing in common—the need for a constant supply of water. These fertile strips form green ribbons throughout the park. Riparian vegetation grows along the four perennial streams that flow through the fold. To a lesser extent, riparian plants line parts of the washes that cut into the fold's tilted rocks. Riparian vegetation can also survive in dry canyons, where runoff waters are concentrated and held in the sands of the washes, and where tall cliffs shelter plants from the desert sun.

Hanging gardens are another highly specialized plant community. These desert oases thrive where springs and seeps issue from protected canyon cliffs. Although hanging gardens are not as abundant in Capitol Reef as they are in more well-watered parks such as Zion, the delicate fronds of maidenhair fern and the colorful blooms of alcove columbine, cardinal flower, and monkey flower provide a beautiful contrast to a backdrop of solid rock and parched desert.

The animal population of Capitol Reef also owes its diversity to the park's varied habitats, though it is not as diverse in numbers as the plant population. The only poisonous reptile in Capitol Reef is the midget faded rattlesnake, a denizen of the slickrock country from east of the High Plateaus in Utah into western Colorado. They are rarely seen in the park, as they blend well into their surroundings, and are quite timid.

The most common reptiles along park trails are the northern plateau and side-blotched lizards; hikers in the Waterpocket District will also encounter sagebrush and desert spiny, leopard, and collared lizards. Short-horned and tree lizards are most common near Fruita and along the Fremont River.

Although Capitol Reef is largely bone-dry slickrock, there is enough water here and there to support a limited number of frogs and toads. The Fremont River is home to the Great Basin spadefoot toad, Rocky Mountain toad, red spotted toad, and leopard frog. The tanks, or waterpockets, and Halls Creek in the Waterpocket District also support these amphibians, as well as the canyon treefrog.

The park is also home to many birds. Some range throughout the park, while others require specialized habitats. The well-developed tree canopy along the Fremont River hosts a wide variety of winged creatures, including yellow and Wilson's warblers, and black-headed grosbeaks. Canyon wrens are denizens of the cliffs and canyons, their descending call unmistakable. The violet-green swallow and white-throated swift are commonly seen flying at high speed among the cliffs in search of their insect prey.

The pinyon-juniper woodlands host the particularly noisy and colorful scrub and pinyon jays. These birds gather in large numbers in autumn if there is an abundant crop of pinyon nuts. The common flicker and yellow-bellied sapsucker also visit wooded areas of the park, whereas the mourning dove, sage thrasher, chukar, western meadowlark, and mockingbird frequent the open desert area east of the fold.

Common nighthawks soar and dive for insects in the evening and early morning hours. American kestrels and sharp-shinned hawks are also soaring birds, but their prey consists of unsuspecting rabbits, squirrels, and mice.

A variety of "little gray birds" also inhabit most areas of the park. Among the more common are the song sparrow, black-throated sparrow, and house finch. Ravens populate most of the park, from the rocky backbone of the fold to the parched desert flats and narrow canyons.

The mule deer is the most obvious and frequently observed large mammal in the park, particularly in the Fruita area. Mountain lions loiter near mule deer, their primary food source. Mountain lion sightings are rare, but a lucky hiker may find the big cat's tracks on a dusty trail or in the mud of a wash. Coyotes are secretive animals, also rarely seen, although their howling and yipping are often heard echoing among the cliffs at night.

Other mammals include the many rodents that inhabit the park. Desert cottontail rabbits and blacktail jackrabbits, which are actually hares rather than rabbits, reside in open desert areas. The whitetail antelope squirrel, which somewhat resembles a chipmunk, is an unmistakable desert dweller, with its tail curled up over its back. Mice are abundant in the park, and though seldom seen, backpackers will likely hear them searching for food in their packs overnight. The desert woodrat, or packrat, is another infrequently seen rodent, although their nests are commonly observed beneath overhanging ledges.

Interpretive activities

Interpretive activities lay the foundation for better understanding and appreciation of Capitol Reef's human and natural history. A stop at the visitor center, located just off Utah Highway 24 at the junction with the park's Scenic Drive, may answer some questions you have about the park, and perhaps whet your appetite to learn more about this historic and unique area. The visitor center offers books and maps for sale, has many interpretive displays featuring plants, geology, and history, and offers a slide program. Rangers on duty can answer your questions on any aspect of the park, and they issue free backcountry use permits to backpackers. The visitor center is open daily, with extended hours in summer.

Evening programs in the Fruita Campground amphitheater are conducted nightly from spring through early fall, and short talks are given in the morning and afternoon. Schedules of activities are posted at the visitor center and campground.

Fruit picking in the Fruita orchards is an important part of a visit to Capitol Reef. Visitors are welcome to stroll through the orchards and eat the ripe fruit, but all fruit must be eaten in the orchards. During the announced harvest periods, visitors may pick all the fruit they wish, for a fee.

Campgrounds

On average, nearly 750,000 visitors come to Capitol Reef each year. Most stay only for a day or less, but those who choose to stay overnight have a variety of campgrounds and motels to choose from in and near the park.

The Fruita Campground lies one mile from the visitor center on the Scenic Drive at an elevation of 5440 feet. The campground lies next to the rushing waters of the Fremont River, and is shaded by broadleaved trees. The campsites, spread across a green lawn, feature picnic tables, fire grills (you must bring your own charcoal and/or wood; wood gathering is not permitted in the park), water, and flush toilets. The campground is open in winter. The fee for camping is charged all year.

The lush, green setting of the campground, surrounded by orchards and historic pioneer buildings, is a startling contrast to the multihued slickrock cliffs and beehive-shaped domes that rear skyward in every direction.

The park has two other campgrounds, in the Cathedral and Waterpocket districts. The Cathedral Campground lies on the flanks of Thousand Lake Mountain at an elevation of 7000 feet, 27.5 miles north of

Utah Highway 24 on the Hartnet Road. No fee is charged at this primitive campground, and campers must bring their own water. There are six campsites nestled in a woodland of pinyon and juniper.

The Cedar Mesa Campground is in the Waterpocket District. It is a beautiful, primitive campground on broad Cedar Mesa at 6000 feet, 21 miles south of Utah Highway 24 on the Notom-Bullfrog Road. A thick woodland shades five campsites, each with a picnic table and fire grill. You must bring your own water. Views southwest into Red Canyon and of the broad mesas east of Waterpocket Fold are superb.

There are several established picnic sites in the park, but visitors are free to picnic anywhere. The large, shady Chestnut and Inglesby picnic areas are located on the Scenic Drive between the visitor center and the Fruita Campground, along the banks of the Fremont River. Other picnic areas are at Capitol Gorge; beside Utah Highway 24, 4.5 miles west of the visitor center; and in the South District beside the Burr Trail road, where one scenic picnic area is atop the fold at the head of the switchbacks above Muley Twist Canyon, and another near the park's western boundary, 29 miles from Boulder.

Several other campgrounds, both public and private, lie close to the park. Three Forest Service campgrounds dot the forested flanks of Boulder Mountain along scenic Utah Highway 12 within 20 miles of the park. Other USFS campgrounds are located near Bicknell and Loa, and there are several others near Fish Lake, high on the Fishlake Plateau 20 miles northwest of Loa, along Utah Highway 24.

Private campgrounds are in Torrey and Hanksville. There are no services available inside the park, but motels, gas, convenience stores, and groceries are available at and near the Utah Highway 12/24 junction 1 mile east of Torrey, and in Torrey, 11 miles west of the visitor center, and Hanksville, 37 miles east of the visitor center, both on Utah 24.

Auto repairs and towing are available in Torrey, Hanksville, Bicknell and Loa. The nearest hospital is 75 miles away in Richfield on U.S. 89, and a medical clinic is in Bicknell, 19 miles west of the visitor center on Utah 24.

Hikers should come to Capitol Reef well equipped, as the nearest source of outdoor supplies is in Richfield.

For more information about Capitol Reef National Park, contact:

Park Superintendent
Capitol Reef National Park
HCR 70 Box 15
Torrey, UT 84775-9602
(435) 425-3791

Hiking in Capitol Reef

Capitol Reef offers some of the finest desert hiking in all of Utah's national parks. All districts offer trails for hikers of every ability, although most are a little more rugged than those in other national parks in Utah.

The Fremont River District, encompassing the rugged Capitol Reef part of Waterpocket fold, is slickrock country at its finest. Bounded by Pleasant Creek on the south and Utah Highway 24 on the north, it contains the greatest concentration of trails. Due to easy access from the highway and paved Scenic Drive, the area receives the most use. Here, along the towering west face of the Waterpocket Fold, trails lead into narrow canyons, traverse mesas and cliffs, and wind among lofty slickrock domes. Trails here are mostly rough and rocky, some are quite steep, and parts of trails cross slickrock where rock cairns must be followed. The trails are well-signed, and can be used to access cross-country routes in canyons and atop the wooded crest of the Waterpocket Fold.

The Waterpocket District, bounded by Utah Highway 24 on the north, by Glen Canyon National Recreation Area on the south, and by Grand Staircase-Escalante National Monument on the west, is accessed via two roads: The Notom-Bullfrog Road, which branches off Utah Highway 24 east of the park, and the Burr Trail Road, heading east from the small town of Boulder on Highway 12. Hiking in the Waterpocket District is largely confined to the numerous slot canyons that penetrate the resistant rocks of the fold. Both roads offer access to these east-west-trending canyons. As in the Fremont River District, there are a few trails here that are fairly easy and are passable to the average hiker. Most hiking routes in this district follow cairns over slickrock or along washes.

For hikers who wish to traverse some of the most isolated and remote desert country in Utah, there's the Cathedral District, north of Utah Highway 24. That district is beyond the scope of this book. Obtain a copy of the author's *Utah's National Parks* (published by Wilderness Press), a comprehensive guidebook that features several backcountry trips in the park's Cathedral District.

Most visitors come to Capitol Reef during summer, when the park experiences its warmest temperatures and when thunderstorms can sweep the Waterpocket Fold, dumping heavy rains, often accompanied by lightning and high winds. July and August are the wettest and hottest months in the park. Temperatures typically reach well into the 90s during summer, and occasionally break 100°. The Waterpocket District is typically warmer than the Headquarters area by at least 5°, and likewise the Cathedral District is usually a bit cooler. The months of April through June and September through November are perhaps the best seasons in which to hike in Capitol Reef—and most other Utah national parks. For more information on hiking seasons, refer to the section "Hiking Utah's desert parks," in the introduction. ■

Hike 14. Chimney Rock Loop Trail

Distance	3.5 miles semiloop trip
Elevation gain	620'
Average hiking time	2 to 2½ hours
Difficulty rating	3
Child rating	2 to 3
Best seasons	April through mid-June; mid-September through November
Hazards	No shade

Driving to the trailhead

Utah Highway 24 is the primary access leading to Capitol Reef National Park, stretching 161 miles from U.S. 89 at Richfield, to Interstate 70 west of Green River. The starting point for the driving directions below is the Utah 24/12 junction, 51 miles west of Hanksville, 66 miles east of Richfield, and and 59 miles north of Escalante.

From the junction of Utah 24 with southbound Utah 12, about 1 mile east of Torrey (the last town encountered eastbound on Utah 24 until Hanksville, some 50 miles distant), follow Utah 24 eastward into Capitol Reef National Park. After 6.8 miles, you reach the signed turnoff to Chimney Rock Trailhead, on the north side of the highway, where a spur leads 50 yards to the parking area.

Introduction

This is a fine half-day hike on a good trail in the western reaches of the park. It offers close-up views of the great barrier cliffs of Capitol Reef, as well as more distant panoramas of the Waterpocket Fold and the high plateaus of Boulder and Thousand Lake mountains. Terrain varies from open flats to a sparsely wooded mesa and a cliffbound canyon.

Description

From the signed Chimney Rock trailhead (6051'), we briefly climb northwest up low red hills of the Moenkopi Formation before leveling off in a grassy flat decorated by scattered shrubs, pinyons, junipers, and a variety of colorful wildflowers from spring through early fall. Chimney Rock rises 400 feet in the southeast, jutting west from the flat mesa above it.

A fascinating pillar composed of Moenkopi rocks, its myriad thin layers are accentuated by weathering and erosion, and they support a single block of tan-colored Shinarump Conglomerate. Such balanced rocks are superb examples of differential erosion, in which rocks of different hardnesses are eroded at different rates. Except for the resistant caprock, Chimney Rock's pillar would be reduced to clay and sand in a comparatively short time.

At the northeast end of the flat, the trail begins a series of steep, short switchbacks that lead upward through the varicolored layers of the Chinle Formation. After this stiff ascent, we reach a signed junction at 0.5 mile (6307') and turn right. To our north the Wingate Sandstone cliffs soar nearly vertically 400 feet, pockmarked by several arch-shaped alcoves. Boulders fallen from these cliffs obscure much of the Chinle Formation below.

Presently ascending north slopes, we soon reach the brink of the Moenkopi cliff and gaze beyond the spire of Chimney Rock to the distant lofty plateau of 11,000-foot Boulder Mountain, where dense forests and unseen, lake-dotted cirque basins form a stark contrast to the comparatively barren, rock-dominated landscape of Capitol Reef. The trail hugs the rim of a Chinle-capped mesa, soon passing a very short spur to an overlook; enroute we enjoy far-flung panoramas of the Henry Mountains to the east, foregrounded by the great red cliffs and white domes of Capitol Reef rising in bold relief. A northeast-trending tributary, Chimney Rock Canyon, slicing deep into the sandstone layers of the reef to our east, is part of the popular but challenging route down Spring Canyon to the Fremont River (see *Utah's National Parks*, by the author). We can also see the dirt road to the Goosenecks Overlook, ending above the deep gorge of Sulphur Creek, south of Utah 24.

Leveling off on the mesa, we pass scattered pinyons and junipers, the live trees gnarled, twisted and stunted by harsh desert winds, growing among the picturesque wind-burnished remains of their predecessors. Soon the trail descends corrugated slopes to a low saddle, then skirts the base of soaring Wingate Sandstone cliffs amid a jumble of large boulders. These red sandstone blocks demonstrate cross-bedding, an indication that this sandstone was deposited by wind. The trail soon descends and bends west down to the nearby signed junction at 2.0 miles (6171'). Here the route into Chimney Rock and Spring canyons heads off to the right, and the return leg of our loop branches left.

We take the left branch, continuing west, and ascend the broad upper drainage of this tributary, with towering red cliffs rising in the north and tree- and shrub-dotted slopes rising gently in the south.

Scattered pinyon and juniper, hop-sage, Mormon Tea, rabbitbrush and a variety of seasonal wildflowers keep us company as we gently ascend slopes and cross the small, dry wash several times. Keep an eye out for petrified wood enroute toward the skyline saddle in the west; it is fairly common in the Chinle Formation. Upon reaching the broad saddle at 2.8 miles (6330'), you can make a brief detour to the south to see more fragments of petrified wood. Remember that collecting is prohibited in the park.

From the saddle we descend north-facing slopes to a junction with the loop trail at 3.0 miles (6307'); we turn right and retrace our panoramic route for 0.5 mile to the trailhead.   ■

Hike 15. Fremont Gorge Viewpoint Trail

Distance	4.4 miles round trip
Elevation gain	1050'
Average hiking time	2½ hours
Difficulty rating	4
Child rating	3
Best seasons	April through mid-June; mid-September through November
Hazards	No shade; steep dropoffs at the trail's end

Driving to the trailhead

See the driving directions for Hike 14 to reach the junction of Utah 24/12. From that junction, about 1 mile east of Torrey (the last town encountered eastbound on Utah 24 until Hanksville, some 50 miles distant), follow Utah 24 eastward into Capitol Reef National Park. After 9.9 miles you reach the southbound turnoff to the park visitor center and the Scenic Drive. Be sure to pick up a copy of the park map at the visitor center before proceeding; it will help you locate starting points for the hiking trails ahead. Follow the Scenic Drive beyond the visitor center for 0.9 mile to the historic Fruita blacksmith shop, on the right (south). Park at either the blacksmith shop or in the parking area a short distance ahead (east), beneath the trees next to the Johnson Orchard.

Introduction

Most trails in Capitol Reef's Fremont River District lead to destinations in the Waterpocket Fold that include narrow canyons, arches, and panoramic overlooks. By contrast, the Fremont Gorge Viewpoint Trail takes hikers in the opposite direction, away from the Waterpocket Fold, to a grand vista point on the rim of a 1000-foot-deep canyon the Fremont River has carved through Miners Mountain. It is one of three trails that leads away from the fold in this part of the park (the Old Wagon and Fremont River trails are the other two). This trail, with a steady uphill grade all the way to the overlook, also affords sweeping vistas of Capitol Reef, and contrasts the rich greenery of the Fruita area with arid mesas and soaring sandstone cliffs.

Description

The hike begins immediately west of the blacksmith shop (5430'), following the road southeast past the locked gate. We ascend a moderate grade across barren, red and gray slopes composed of the Chinle Formation. The grade eases as we curve around the east point of Johnson Mesa, directly above shady Chestnut Picnic Area. As the road begins a southwest-bound traverse, the foot trail branches right (west) at 0.2 mile, where a sign indicates FREMONT GORGE VIEWPOINT-1.8 (actual mileage is 2.0).

Follow the good, wide trail as it carves a pair of switchbacks, then rises very steeply to the edge of Johnson Mesa, where the grade becomes gentle. Black volcanic boulders mantle the landscape of the mesa, sharing space with a sparse covering of bunchgrasses, shadscale, snakeweed, and green Torrey ephedra (Mormon Tea). Vistas open up as we follow the southeast rim of the mesa, stretching past the historic Gifford Farm to the verdant campground below us to the south, and to cottonwood-bordered Sulphur Creek and the Johnson Orchard to the north. Directly below, the rock fence built long ago by Cal Pendleton, an early Fruita settler, follows a sinuous course southwest along the lower slopes of the mesa.

Superb views from the open, shadeless mesa stretch along the bold cliffs of the Waterpocket Fold from Thousand Lake Mountain in the northwest toward Pleasant Creek far to the southeast, and reach eastward down the dome-bounded canyon of the Fremont River. As we progress toward the southwest reaches of the mesa, pinyon and juniper begin to stud the trailside slopes. Soon after entering the woodland the mesa blends into slopes of red Moenkopi Formation rocks that tilt upward toward the west.

Once we reach the red slopes, the trail curves into a shallow wooded draw flanked by low redrock cliffs. Heading toward a prominent red knob, the trail leaves the draw and we ascend a steady, moderate grade. The grade grows steep as we rise past the knob and top out on the canyon rim just above it. The trail ahead leaves the rim and continues to rise steeply over rubbly, tan-colored Moenkopi rocks. Only the south wall of Fremont Gorge is visible as we make our way upward through an open woodland.

Up and up the trail climbs, until we finally reach a large cairn on the canyon rim at 2.2 miles (6480'), where a tremendous view opens up into the labyrinth below. The red rocks of the Moenkopi Formation cap the canyon rims 800 to 1000 feet above the gorge. Below are terraced cliff bands composed of the light gray rocks of Kaibab Limestone and White Rim Sandstone—the oldest rocks exposed in Capitol Reef. The Fremont River can be heard, but not seen, as it flows through a narrow, sinuous inner gorge far below.

The rugged gorge frames a fine view of lofty Boulder Mountain to the southwest, while behind us are vistas of Johnson Mesa, now lying far below,

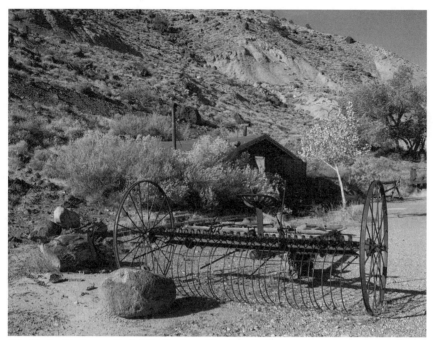

The blacksmith shop at Capitol Reef is the trailhead for the Fremont Gorge Viewpoint Trail

and beyond it the Fruita Campground spreads out beneath the colorful cliffs of the Waterpocket Fold. More distant views include broad Horse Mesa on the northeast skyline above the lower Fremont River canyon; Mounts Ellen and Pennell in the Henry Mountains, on the southeast horizon beyond the dome-crowned crest of the Waterpocket Fold; and far away, beyond distant mesas and plateaus, the La Sal Mountains near Moab.

From the viewpoint, retrace your steps to the trailhead. ∎

Hike 16. Fremont River Trail

Distance	2.5 miles round trip
Elevation gain	465'
Average hiking time	1 to 1½ hours
Difficulty rating	2
Child rating	1 for the first 0.5 mile; 2 thereafter
Best seasons	April through mid-June; mid-September through November
Hazards	No shade; steep dropoffs

Driving to the trailhead

See the driving directions for Hike 14 to reach the Utah 24/12 junction. From that junction, about 1 mile east of Torrey (the last town encountered eastbound on Utah 24 until Hanksville, some 50 miles distant), follow Utah 24 eastward into Capitol Reef National Park. After 9.9 miles you reach the southbound turnoff to the park visitor center and the Scenic Drive. Be sure to pick up a copy of the park map at the visitor center before proceeding; it will help you locate starting points for the hiking trails ahead.

Hikers have a choice of three starting points for the Fremont River Trail: 1) park at the Chestnut or Inglesby picnic areas, 1 mile from the visitor center on the Scenic Drive, and find the trail on the south side of the Fremont River bridge next to the Gifford farmhouse. 2) Park at the Cohab Canyon Trailhead, immediately east of the Gifford barn. 3) Drive 1.5 miles from the visitor center and enter Campground Loop C, signed for the amphitheater and group area. Park in the amphitheater parking area at the west end of the campground loop, and begin hiking there.

Introduction

From the historic Fruita orchards to the commanding vista point at the trail's end, this fine hike captures the essence of the Capitol Reef experience, contrasting the Fremont River's ribbon of green with arid mesas, and the manicured lawns of the campground and the neat rows of the orchards with a chaotic jumble of towering slickrock domes and sheer cliffs. Seven sedimentary layers stretch 250 million years into the past represent the earth's geologic history.

The initial riverside segment of the trail is gravelled, and it is the only handicap-accessible trail in the park.

Description

The signed trail begins on the Scenic Drive next to the Gifford farmhouse, or at the west end of Campground Loop B (5435'), and follows the east bank of the river upstream between apple and pear orchards on the left, and wildrose thickets and the unusually tall common reed grass on the right. Wildlife abounds in the orchards of Fruita: mule deer, marmots, skunks, and beavers are particularly common. Park managers have installed protective coverings around the trunks of trees here to save them from cambium-eating beavers, while the abundant mule deer enjoy eating not only the lush grasses in the orchards but also the trees' leaves and bark. Many of Fruita's orchards are encircled by tall "deer proof" fences.

The boulders of the fence across the river and those that litter Johnson Mesa and much of Capitol Reef, especially in the Fremont River canyon, originated from the lava fields atop Boulder and Thousand Lake mountains. These boulders, which are either round or angular, were once thought to have been carried here by swiftly running streams and rivers that drained melting high-country glaciers thousands of years ago. New studies show that the boulders were transported from the mountains in cement-like debris flows, or landslides, filling the ancient valley of the Fremont River. Erosion has since downcut the river valley, leaving the boulders presently high above on river terraces.

The wide, gravel-surfaced trail, accessible to wheelchairs for 0.5 mile, quite soon passes the campground amphitheater. Wedged between a peach orchard and the tumultuous waters of the Fremont, we soon pass a fenced-in smokehouse and sorghum mill, and reach the path joining on our left from the amphitheater parking area in Campground Loop C. Here another sign identifies our route as the Fremont River Trail, and informative pamphlets describing the trail are available from a dispenser. We then pass one more orchard, this one supporting apricot trees, skirt a grassy meadow on our left, and soon reach a fenceline.

Here the gravel surface ends, the trail narrows, and we soon rise moderately upon northwest-facing slopes below red ledges of the Moenkopi Formation. Climbing past the various layers of the Moenkopi, our trail bends southeast, traversing above a precipitous Fremont tributary canyon. Two switchbacks ensue, leading us above a thin, yellowish rock layer—the Sinbad Limestone—one of the five units of the Moenkopi in the park. Shortly we reach the overlook at the trail's end at 1.25 miles (5900'). Toward the southwest, the yawning gorge of the Fremont cuts deeply into a wooded plateau, separating westward-rising Miners Mountain on the south from broad Beas Lewis Flats on the north. The most extensive outcrops of the park's most ancient rock, the White Rim Sandstone, lie exposed in the depths of the canyon.

From northwest to southeast, we can view much of the western facade of Capitol Reef, the most dramatic part of the vast Waterpocket Fold. Eastward, on the face of Capitol Reef, we can see five varicolored rock formations rising from the campground to the skyline—the red Moenkopi, the gray, green and maroon Chinle Formation, the towering orange-red cliffs of the Wingate Sandstone, the wooded benches of the Kayenta Formation, and finally the whitish cliffs and domes of the Navajo Sandstone. The rugged aspect of Capitol Reef contrasts dramatically with the orchards and lush greenery of the river bottom. On the horizon from northwest to southwest, the extensive plateaus of Boulder and Thousand Lake mountains, with their cool, subalpine forests, aspen thickets, and flower-filled meadows, look particularly inviting on a blistering hot summer day.

From the viewpoint, we retrace our steps to the trailhead. ■

Hike 17. Grand Wash

Distance	4.4 miles round trip
Elevation loss	200'
Average hiking time	1 to 1½ hours
Difficulty rating	2
Child rating	2
Best seasons	April through mid-June; mid-September through November
Hazards	Route is rough and rocky; flash-flood danger

Driving to the trailhead

See driving directions for Hike 15 to reach the Capitol Reef visitor center and the Scenic Drive. Follow the Scenic Drive generally southeast past the Fruita Historical District and the campground. After paying the park entrance fee at the self-pay fee station just beyond the campground, continue following the narrow, winding, but paved Scenic Drive. After driving 3.5 miles from the visitor center, turn left (northeast) onto the signed Grand Wash road. Follow this dirt road for another 1.2 miles to the trailhead.

Introduction

Grand Wash is one of only six drainages that begin west of the Waterpocket Fold and flow through it. The hike down the wash is a delightful stroll for hikers of every ability, featuring nearly vertical sandstone walls rising 600-800 feet from the wash and ending in great sky-piercing crags. In a short but memorable narrows the canyon floor is barely 16 feet wide. Signs at the upper and lower trailheads warn that hikers should not enter the canyon when there is a threat of thunderstorms.

Description

The trailhead (5400'), lies in the shadow of immense orange Wingate Sandstone cliffs. We begin our journey here by treading the short trail to the wash bottom, where we proceed down-canyon beneath an imposing dome.

The large tributary of Bear Canyon joins on our right (southeast) soon after we leave the trailhead and stretches up to the crest of the Waterpocket Fold. It is worthy of exploration if time and energy allow.

Shortly beyond Bear Canyon we meet the southern terminus of the Frying Pan Trail at 0.2 mile (5380'), and continue straight ahead down the wash. Unlike many sandy washes in the park, Grand Wash has a hard-packed surface that allows easy progress. This dry wash is occasionally swept by flash floods, which eradicate any colonizing riparian vegetation. Instead of riparian trees, vegetation in the wash is typical of the park's pinyon-juniper woodland: singleleaf ash, big sagebrush, squawbush, rabbitbrush, Utah serviceberry, and cliffrose. In addition, a variety of colorful wildflowers in season adorns the nearly barren slickrock canyon.

At 1.0 mile from the trailhead we enter The Narrows, a claustrophobic 0.5-mile stretch where the wash is about 16 feet wide, hemmed in by cliffs soaring abruptly as much as 800 feet from the canyon floor. Stained by desert varnish, prominently cross-bedded, and dimpled with solution cavities, these high-angle Navajo Sandstone cliffs begin to diminish in stature as we exit The Narrows, and they become progressively lower as we amble out onto Utah Highway 24 at 2.2 miles (5200'), deep within the Fremont River canyon.

From there, retrace your route to the trailhead. ■

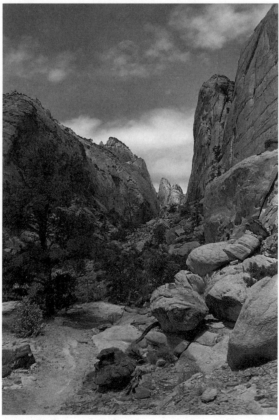

Grand Wash

Hike 18. Old Wagon Trail

Distance	4.0 miles semiloop trip
Elevation gain	1030'
Average hiking time	2 to 2½ hours
Difficulty rating	4
Child rating	3
Best seasons	April through mid-June; mid-September through November
Hazards	Little shade; trail is rough and rocky in places

Driving to the trailhead

Follow driving directions for Hikes 14 and 15 to reach the Capitol Reef visitor center and the Scenic Drive. Follow the Scenic Drive past the visitor center and through the Fruita Historical District, and continue driving southeast along the foot of the Waterpocket Fold.

From the junction with the Grand Wash spur road, 3.5 miles from the visitor center, continue southeast on the Scenic Drive. After another 2.5 miles, the road tops out on Slickrock Divide, then descends toward Capitol Gorge. The signed OLD WAGON TRAIL HIKERS PARKING area is on the right (west) side of the road 0.6 mile from Slickrock Divide, and 6.6 miles from the visitor center.

Introduction

Much like the Fremont Gorge Viewpoint Trail (Hike 15), the Old Wagon Trail leads hikers away from the Waterpocket Fold and onto the slopes of Miners Mountain. The rewards of the stiff climb through the pinyon-juniper woodlands are superb views of the heart of the rugged Waterpocket Fold—Capitol Reef.

Description

From the trailhead (5870'), look westward up the steadily rising, heavily wooded slopes of Miners Mountain. Punctuating the slopes is a small, red- and tan-colored butte. Our trail will lead us to a fine vista point atop that butte, and we get started behind the hikers parking sign by dropping over a ledge of Moenkopi Formation rocks via steps. We quickly reach a shallow wash where a sign indicates the OLD WAGON ROAD LOOP TRAIL.

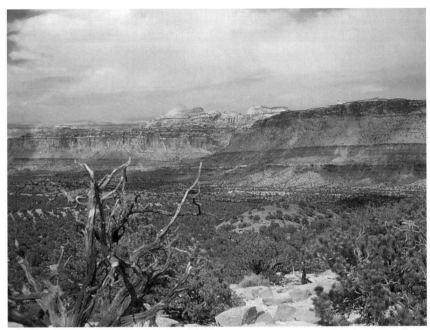

Broad vistas of Capitol Reef unfold from the Old Wagon Trail

From the wash the trail leads westward on a steady ascent of Miners Mountain, through a woodland of pinyon and juniper and over redrock slopes, staying at first just south of the rim of a shallow draw. Gnarled pinyons and junipers are scattered across the slopes, the spaces between them supporting shrubs including sagebrush, snakeweed, Utah serviceberry, cliffrose, buffaloberry, and single-leaf ash.

Soon we mount red Moenkopi slickrock, where cairns guide us first southwest, then west on a steady uphill grade. Spreading out from northwest to southeast are the multicolored cliffs of the Waterpocket Fold, and as we gain elevation massive Mount Ellen, highest of the Henry Mountains, comes into view in the southeast beyond the cleft of Capitol Gorge. The grade is steady enough that we will likely pause often to catch our breath and to enjoy the vistas that continue to expand as we ascend.

After gaining 600 feet in 1.1 miles, we reach the junction with the loop trail, where a trailside post directs us onto the left- branching leg of the loop, leading us southwest in a clockwise direction. The trail ahead is rough and rocky, winding a way upward over the rubbly tan sandstone of the Moenkopi Formation. At length we approach the rim of a prominent, west-trending canyon—Capitol Wash. In its depths we can see the gray rocks of the Kaibab Limestone, the same formation that caps the rims of the Grand Canyon.

Soon the grade abates as we bend northwest and traverse through the woodland on the very rocky trail to the track of the old wagon road, cutting an extremely rocky swath to the east and west and leading straight up and down the flanks of Miners Mountain. Little is known about the origins of this rugged "road," but it reportedly cut through Capitol Gorge and Miners Mountain as a route between Old Highway 24 and the flanks of Boulder Mountain.

Here another trailside post directs us briefly eastward down the rocky wagon road for a few hundred yards, then the trail leads us north away from the rocky swath to a low saddle at 2.0 miles (6800'). A sign here points to the viewpoint (on the butte we saw from the trailhead), and the round-trip hike to it is only 0.1 mile. We head north, then east on this spur trail, and after a few hundred yards we mount tan Moenkopi slabs, where the finest vistas on the trail unfold. Enjoy the vast panoramas of the Waterpocket Fold, Thousand Lake Mountain, and the Henry Mountains before backtracking to the junction, where yet another post points toward the trailhead.

Heading southeast, downhill, our trail leads across the old wagon track, then along a winding course for 0.8 mile, to where we return to our inbound trail. We close the loop there and then turn left (east), backtracking 1.1 miles to the trailhead. ■

Hike 19. Capitol Gorge Trailhead to The Tanks

Distance	1.8 miles round trip
Elevation gain	40'
Average hiking time	1 hour
Difficulty rating	2
Child rating	1
Best seasons	April through mid-June; mid-September through November
Hazards	flash-flood danger

Driving to the trailhead

Follow driving directions for Hikes 14 and 15 to reach the Capitol Reef visitor center and the Scenic Drive. Follow the Scenic Drive past the visitor center and through the Fruita Historical District, and continue driving southeast along the foot of the Waterpocket Fold. After 7.9 miles from the visitor center, you reach the end of pavement and a junction. Continue straight ahead at the junction, following the dirt Capitol Gorge Road for 2.2 miles to the trailhead and picnic area.

Introduction

Capitol Gorge is a narrow defile cut deeply into the Navajo Sandstone of the Waterpocket Fold, and hikers there feel as if they were in a great, yawning cleft deep within the earth. Capitol Gorge probably formed as running water eroded along a joint, or crack, in the fold, deepening the canyon but scarcely widening it. Fremont Indians left their mysterious petroglyphs on the canyon walls, and inscriptions of early travelers can also be found along the old road.

A hike through Capitol Gorge to The Tanks is a delightful stroll for hikers of every ability, and it allows one to contemplate the evolution of slickrock canyons, the mysterious Fremont rock artists, and the pioneers and early settlers who built and used this old "road" through a precipitous, flood-prone canyon.

Description

The trailhead (5400') lies in the shadow of immense cliffs of Navajo Sandstone, and from here we proceed along the former route of Utah Highway 24. After 0.2 mile we reach the petroglyphs (rock carvings), just beyond the point where the Kayenta Formation beds have dipped underground. One of only two easily accessible Fremont petroglyphs in the park, it consists of a group of broad-shouldered human-like figures without arms, wearing head-dresses of feathers or curved horns. Unfortunately, here as in many other places in the gorge, modern-day "graffiti artists" have defiled the petroglyphs with their carvings.

Quite soon the old road disappears and we proceed through a memorable narrows, where great desert-varnished cliffs loom above. At 0.5 mile is the Pioneer Register, where travelers following Elijah Behunin's "Blue Dugway" through the fold left signs of their passing. The earliest carvings on the walls here date back to 1871, when a "JA. Call" and "Wal. Bateman," early prospectors, passed through the gorge hoping to find gold. Many other inscriptions date back to the late 19th century but are confused among myriad modern-day carvings and bullet holes. Numerous iron rods protruding from the canyon walls are remnants of a telephone line that served early settlements east of the fold.

After another 0.5 mile through the narrow, tortuous canyon, a sign indicates The Tanks (5360'), 1.0 mile from the trailhead (actual mileage is 0.9), which lie just above the wash at the mouth of an inconspicuous west-trending canyon. These large waterpockets can be reached by scrambling up the slickrock at the canyon's juncture with Capitol Gorge. They hold a great deal of water, particularly after heavy rains and in spring, and are an important source of moisture for Capitol Reef wildlife. Look for a small natural bridge at The Tanks.

Just 100 yards down-canyon, fascinating Waterpocket Canyon leads off to our right (southeast), draining the apex of the fold. A trail of sorts leads briefly up the sandy mouth of the canyon, soon disappearing in the slickrock. Adventurous and experienced hikers will find this steep canyon, with its narrows and its numerous waterpockets, an exciting route for attaining the crest of the fold. Downstream, the canyon walls diminish in height as Capitol Wash winds its way another 1.5 miles to the park boundary and to the Notom-Bullfrog Road beyond. Most hikers will turn around at The Tanks and backtrack to the trailhead. ■

Hike 20. Golden Throne Trail

Distance	4.0 miles round trip
Elevation gain	700'
Average hiking time	2 to 2½ hours
Difficulty rating	4
Child rating	3
Best seasons	April through mid-June; mid-September through November
Hazards	Little shade; steep dropoffs

Driving to the trailhead

Follow driving directions for Hike 19.

Introduction

Golden Throne is one of the premier slickrock domes in Capitol Reef. This golden-toned butte dominates the view from many remote corners of the park, its smooth cliffs jutting skyward 600 feet above its surroundings. This scenic trail offers access from Capitol Gorge to the top of the Waterpocket Fold, where hikers gain a head-on view of Golden Throne, and more distant panoramas that stretch from the Henry Mountains in the east to the wooded slope of Miners Mountain in the west.

Description

From Capitol Gorge Trailhead (5400') turn left on the rocky trail and climb west beneath an overhanging ledge of Kayenta Sandstone. The trail soon bends into and out of three interesting side canyons high above Capitol Gorge, where spectacular views reach into the dome-capped heart of Capitol Reef.

Curving into the third in this series of small canyons after 1 mile, we gain our first glimpse of Golden Throne. Its sheer southeast face, desert-varnished and stained a golden color by its cap of reddish Carmel Formation rocks, thrusts skyward over 1300 feet above us. Its flat crown, studded with gnarled pinyons and junipers, forms a striking contrast to its smooth, golden cliffs, a scene typical of the Colorado Plateau, where sheer cliffs seem universally to edge nearly horizontal beds. Golden Throne is a butte, the erosional remnant of a mesa, which in turn is the erosional remnant of a more vast surface called a plateau.

Ahead, gnarled, weather-beaten pinyons and junipers dot the rocky ledges. Many of them are barely clinging to existence, nurtured through only a single strip of bark. With their counterparts that have succumbed to the harsh environment, they provide foreground for constant inspiring vistas of the vertical world of Capitol Reef.

After switchbacking up and away from this side canyon, we cross over a low ridge and contour northwest, greeted by a view of the imposing plateau of Boulder Mountain in the west, foregrounded by the gentle, densely wooded slopes of Miners Mountain. South along the crest of the fold, the subdued, ledgy landscape composed of Kayenta rocks, tree-clad and punctuated by myriad erosional forms, contrasts with the domes and cliffs that dominate our view east of the crest.

Presently the trail climbs easily, contouring briefly into yet another minor canyon before curving south to its terminus at a fine viewpoint at 2.0 miles (6100'). From here we can gaze into the abyss of Capitol Gorge, beyond which the dome-capped fold frames a grand view of the Henry Mountains to the east. The bronze sentinel of Golden Throne, however, captures our attention, jutting nearly 1000 feet into the Utah sky to the north only 0.5 mile from our viewpoint.

From the viewpoint, retrace your steps to the trailhead. ■

Hike 21. Hickman Bridge Trail

Distance	1.9 miles round trip
Elevation gain	320'
Average hiking time	1 to 1½ hours
Difficulty rating	2
Child rating	2
Best seasons	April through mid-June; mid-September through November
Hazards	Negligible

Driving to the trailhead

Follow driving directions for Hikes 14 and 15 to reach the Capitol Reef visitor center, then continue east on Utah 24 for 2 miles to the signed Hickman Bridge trailhead parking area.

Introduction

The Hickman Bridge Trail is one of the most popular trails in Capitol Reef. This fairly easy hike surveys a variety of park scenery, ranging from the sandy, cottonwood-lined banks of the Fremont River to arid benches littered with volcanic boulders, to a slickrock canyon bounded by soaring sandstone domes, and finally to the most famous natural rock span in the park.

The trail is easy to follow but little shade is available enroute. Eighteen numbered posts along the way are keyed to a trail guide available at the trailhead or at the visitor center.

Description

From the trailhead (5330') we proceed east under a broken red cliff composed of Kayenta Formation rocks, following along the north bank of the turbulent river. Presently we find ourselves in a riparian environment, where water-dependent Fremont cottonwoods, tamarisk, and willows thrive.

Our jaunt along the verdant Fremont River oasis abruptly ends and we switchback up southeast-facing slopes, entering the arid environment that predominates in Capitol Reef. This sun-drenched ascent is decorated by sparse grasses, the orange springtime blooms of globe mallow, and desert-varnished volcanic boulders. At 0.3 mile (5470') we arrive at a junction with the right-forking, northbound Rim Overlook/Navajo Knobs Trail, leading to aerial-like vistas high above Fruita. Eastward is a memorable head-on view of Capitol Dome, the namesake of the park, visible since the trailhead.

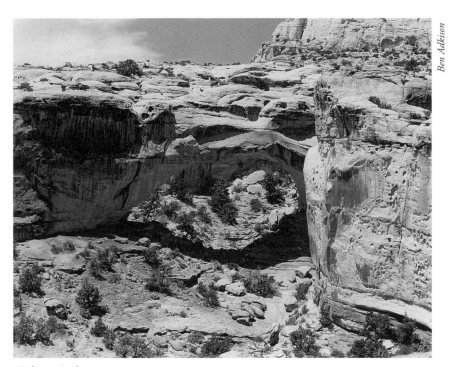

Hickman Bridge

From the junction we continue straight ahead (west) toward Hickman Bridge. We steadily ascend an open slope strewn with dark volcanic boulders deposited by ancient landslides from their source atop Thousand Lake and Boulder mountains. Soon we descend briefly to the banks of a minor sandy wash. Working our way westward along the south banks of the wash, we reach the opening of Nels Johnson Bridge spanning the wash, named for one of the earliest homesteaders in the Fruita area.

Just beyond, the trail splits at 0.8 mile (5600'), forming a loop under and around Hickman Bridge. Bearing right we traverse pinyon- and juniper-dotted slickrock above the wash. Soon the trail leads up to and through Hickman Bridge at 0.9 mile (5650'), one of the largest spans in the park, with dimensions of 125 feet top to bottom by 133 feet between abutments. The bulk of the bridge is formed in the tan sandstones of the Kayenta, while its abutments rest on the softer red mudstones of the same formation. Differential weathering in which softer rocks below broke down faster than those above contributed to the spalling off of rock slabs: where the once-supportive basal rocks were removed, it hastened the formation of an alcove and ultimately an arch. Some geologists believe Hickman Bridge to actually be an arch whose opening pre-dated the formation of the shallow wash that presently courses beneath it. If this is correct, it is reasonable to assume that the present-day drainage has, at the least, contributed to the enlargement of the opening.

A favorite of late-afternoon photographers, Hickman Bridge frames some of the most inspiring scenery in Capitol Reef; a chaotic jumble of white domes and desert-varnished cliffs etched into the Utah sky combine to make the scene one of unforgettable, compelling beauty.

After passing through the great rock opening, the trail curves southeast through hummocky slickrock. After about 250 yards, a very short spur trail forks right, offering a fine view of the Fremont River. The main trail then leads northeast to the aforementioned junction at 1.1 miles (5600'), whence we retrace our route for 0.8 mile to the trailhead. ■

Hike 22. Rim Overlook/Navajo Knobs Trail

Distance	9.0 miles round trip
Elevation gain	1,650'
Average hiking time	5 hours
Difficulty rating	5
Child rating	3
Best seasons	April through mid-June; mid-September through November
Hazards	Steep dropoffs; no shade

Driving to the trailhead

Follow driving directions for Hike 21.

Introduction

Rim Overlook, perched atop the sheer cliffs that soar skyward north of Fruita and Utah Highway 24, offers a commanding, unobstructed vista of the rugged reaches of Capitol Reef. An even more comprehensive, 360° panorama unfolds from Navajo Knobs at the trail's end, atop the sandstone knobs perched on the rim of the Waterpocket Fold.

This rigorous trail climbs steadily from the Fremont River, crossing much slickrock enroute. Hikers should make the effort to follow the cairns across slickrock between Rim Overlook and Navajo Knobs, instead of crossing soil-covered areas that support easily-crushed cryptobiotic crust. Allow ample time to absorb the vista and perhaps to explore the hanging canyons between Rim Overlook and Navajo Knobs.

Description

From the Hickman Bridge trailhead follow Hike 20 for 0.3 mile to the junction (5470') with the Hickman Bridge Trail. Our trail forks off to the right (north), passing among erratic volcanic boulders enroute toward desert-varnished Navajo Sandstone cliffs soaring 500 feet skyward. Quite soon we briefly descend to cross a dry wash and then curve northwest for a climb up along it.

Climbing away from the wash beneath striking cliffs, we reach the Hickman Bridge View Point at 0.8 mile (5670'). Pause here to walk out on the sandstone point for an intriguing view of Hickman Bridge, spanning the wash below to the southwest.

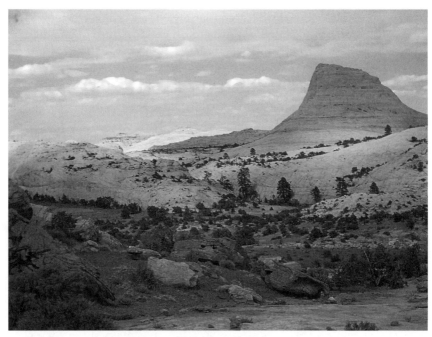

Domes surround Longleaf Flat near the Navajo Knobs Trail

Above us to our north, Kayenta rocks, which our trail presently crosses, give way to what many consider the most notable rock formation in the park—the Navajo Sandstone—which has a typical ridgeline aspect of hummocky domes, abutted by smooth cliffs featuring a tapestry of desert varnish on their faces.

Ahead we curve into and out of two box canyons, the second of which drains under Hickman Bridge. After climbing moderately out of the second wash, we pass through abundant dune sand, anchored by scattered trees and shrubs. This sand has collected below the Navajo cliffs, which themselves are former dune sand that was cemented into stone in ancient times and once again is weathering into its parent material.

Ahead we bend into and out of two more dry drainages and cross abundant slickrock, where cairns help guide us. Beyond the fourth draw, we finally reach Rim Overlook at 2.3 miles (6375'), precariously perched atop sheer cliffs plunging nearly 1000 feet toward the confluence of Sulphur Creek and the Fremont River. Our dramatic aerial-like view takes in Utah Highway 24, the Fruita Campground, and the scattered Fruita orchards. We can trace the park's Scenic Drive as it heads southeast through a deep red badlands landscape beneath the sheer west facade of the Waterpocket Fold.

The sloping, densely wooded mesa of Miners Mountain rises west of the Scenic Drive, while the crest of forest-topped Boulder Mountain forms a horizon beyond. Eastward, the deep, narrow chasm of the Fremont River meanders among the mammoth domes of the fold, forming a picturesque frame for the vast San Rafael Desert stretching eastward to the horizon. Other isolated mountain ranges meet our gaze in the heat-hazy distance beyond: the second highest mountains in Utah—the La Sals—punctuate the northeast horizon 110 miles distant, while a sliver of the Abajo Mountains peeks above the crest of the Henrys, 100 miles to the southeast.

From the overlook hikers can either return to the trailhead or strike out north along the cairned trail to Navajo Knobs, 2.2 miles ahead. The trail continues traversing the sloping Kayenta ledge beyond Rim Overlook, leading north-northwest into the draw immediately south of the sandy and grassy, tree-studded expanse of Longleaf Flat. A boot-worn path leads north from the draw toward the flat, amid Navajo domes shaded by pinyon and juniper and a few large ponderosa pines. Hikers must avoid trampling the abundant, fragile cryptobiotic crust in Longleaf Flat.

From the draw the trail ascends the slickrock bench southwest past a small stand of ponderosa pines. Fine views from the bench reach northeast into the dome-encircled openings of Longleaf Flat. We rise over slickrock at a moderate grade, soon curving around a point a short distance north of a small radio antenna. As we begin a descending, northbound traverse of the Kayenta ledge, views open up to reveal the splintered Wingate Sandstone butte of The Castle, resting on a foundation of colorful Chinle Formation badlands slopes below to the west.

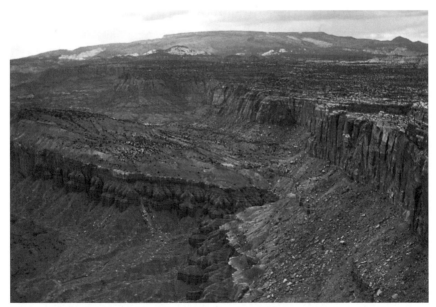

Mummy Cliffs and Thousand Lake Mountain from Navajo Knobs

Our traverse proceeds downhill, following the dip of the Waterpocket Fold's rock beds. Ahead we can visually trace our route along the ledge, first north, then west, to the Navajo Knobs, which rise on the west end of the point northwest of The Castle. Our trail, mostly a cairned route across Kayenta slickrock, passes beneath a desert-varnished wall of Navajo Sandstone. Wherever soil has collected in this rockbound landscape, gnarled pinyons and junipers stud the landscape, sharing space with such shrubs as buffaloberry and littleleaf mountain mahogany.

The traverse eventually leads us past a series of four small, boulder-choked draws; we then curve southwest, following cairns that lead us on a moderate- to-steep uphill grade. This is a sustained uphill grind, but it provides fine stretches of slickrock walking, and memorable vistas of the Navajo Sandstone domes that crown the Waterpocket Fold.

The steep grade abates when we curve into a rockbound draw. Just ahead rise the Navajo Knobs, capping the end of the next point on the rim of the fold. The trail soon grows steep again as we wind our way along the final several yards to the southern foot of the knobs. From there we mount Navajo Sandstone slickrock, and ascend a steep, rocky, sandy stretch to the summit of the knobs at 4.5 miles (6979').

The vistas, perhaps the finest from any point reached by a trail in the park, are far-ranging and panoramic. Far below, Utah Highway 24 winds westward across a redrock landscape, and we also see the Goosenecks Overlook Road stretching to the rim of cavernous Sulphur Creek canyon. Below to the west are the red Mummy Cliffs, beyond which the orange face of the Waterpocket Fold stretches northwest and eventually blends into the gentle slopes of Thousand Lake Mountain. Miles of knobby slickrock, colored orange and white and studded with woodlands of pinyon and juniper, stretch north of the rim of the fold. Far to the east, beyond the slickrock landscape of Capitol Reef, colorful badlands hills, mesas, and buttes stretch into the distant San Rafael Desert. Most prominent is towering Factory Butte.

The Henry Mountains thrust their massive flanks skyward in the southeast. Far below to the south are the Fruita orchards and the visitor center. Above that verdant oasis we see the tilted rock beds of the fold in profile, stretching to the southeast. West of the fold our view reaches up the sloping, wooded flanks of Miners Mountain, and past the gorges of Sulphur Creek and the Fremont River, where the ancient gray rocks of the Kaibab Limestone are exposed. On the southwest skyline beyond are the broad slopes of Boulder Mountain, mantled in oak, aspen, and conifer forests beneath its lofty volcanic rim. Finally, our westward view reaches far up the Fremont River valley to the distant Awapa Plateau on the western horizon.

From Navajo Knobs, retrace your route to the trailhead. ∎

Hike 23. Surprise Canyon

Distance	2 miles round trip
Elevation gain	230'
Average hiking time	1 to 1½ hours
Difficulty rating	3
Child rating	3
Best seasons	April through mid-June; mid-September through November
Hazards	Some scrambling required; flash-flood danger

Driving to the trailhead

Surprise Canyon, and nearby Headquarters Canyon, are located in the remote southern reaches of the park's Waterpocket District. To get there, hikers can follow either the Notom-Bullfrog Road or the Burr Trail Road.

To find the Notom-Bullfrog Road, see driving directions for Hikes 14 and 15 to reach the Capitol Reef visitor center, then continue east on Utah 24 for another 9 miles to the prominently signed turnoff, and proceed south on the two-lane pavement of the Notom-Bullfrog Road. The pavement ends after 5 miles, and thereafter the dirt road is often rough, but usually passable to passenger vehicles, in dry weather only. Heavy rainfall can make this road impassable even to 4WD vehicles, and flash floods may wash out the road in places. The drive to the trailhead is long and slow, but very scenic.

After driving 32.7 miles south from Utah 24, you reach a major junction with the westbound Burr Trail Road. That road begins on Utah 12 in the town of Boulder and leads 36.3 miles to this junction. The road is paved through Grand Staircase- Escalante National Monument for 30.5 miles to the west boundary of the park, the remaining 5.8 miles being a rough and rocky dirt road.

From that junction, continue southeast on the Notom-Bullfrog Road for 1.7 miles to the signed Surprise Canyon hikers parking area on the right (west) side of the road.

Introduction

Untold dozens of narrow slot canyons cut deeply into the Waterpocket Fold in the park's Waterpocket District. In order to ascend through most of these canyons, some wading and even swimming of deep potholes and some rock climbing may be necessary, making them accessible only to seasoned canyoneers. But the short hikes into Surprise and nearby Headquarters

canyons (Hike 24) are open to most any hiker, and offer a tantalizing introduction to the slickrock slot canyons of the Waterpocket Fold. If a thunderstorm is brewing over the fold, save the hikes in these canyons for another
day.

Description

From the trailhead (4900'), where a sliver of Peak-a-boo Rock can be
viewed atop the fold in the northwest, our sandy trail heads southwest, crosses a shallow gully, and proceeds across greasewood-clad flats. Fine over-the-
shoulder views extend east across the valley of Halls Creek to sandstone-
capped mesas rising above barren Mancos Shale slopes. As we head toward
the warped strata of the Waterpocket Fold, here dominated by glistening
white Navajo Sandstone, a series of narrow, forbidding chasms gives only a
vague suggestion of hidden passageways into the depths of that great barrier.

At 0.2 mile we reach the usually dry, tamarisk-lined wash of Halls
Creek. Beyond it we climb over a bunchgrass- and juniper-dotted hill via the
sandy trail, after which we descend into the wash of Surprise Canyon, where
the trail ends at 0.4 mile, amid dwarf clumps of wavy-leaf oak. Ascending
the dry course of the wash, we see that red hills of the Carmel Formation
give way to sky-piercing cliffs of Navajo Sandstone, topped by striking pinnacles and crags.

The Navajo cliffs, rising as much as 600 feet nearly vertically from the
canyon bottom, are encrusted with green, gray and black lichens, as well as
brown, black and metallic-blue desert varnish. After almost one mile, the
sandy, rock-littered wash narrows considerably. Cliffs are ever higher as we
proceed, and we soon reach an interesting undercut and an extremely narrow cleft, where the canyon squeezes down to an opening mere inches wide
at 1.0 mile (5100').

Return the way you came. ■

Hike 24. Headquarters Canyon

Distance	3.0 miles round trip
Elevation gain	560'
Average hiking time	1½ to 2 hours
Difficulty rating	3
Child rating	3
Best seasons	April through mid-June; mid-September through November
Hazards	Flash-flood danger

Driving to the trailhead

Follow driving directions for Hike 23 to the Surprise Canyon Trailhead, and continue southeast on the Notom-Bullfrog Road for 0.5 mile to the signed Headquarters Canyon hikers parking area.

Introduction

This short but fascinating jaunt into a narrow slot canyon is much like the trip into Surprise Canyon. In the late 19th century, the trailhead was a

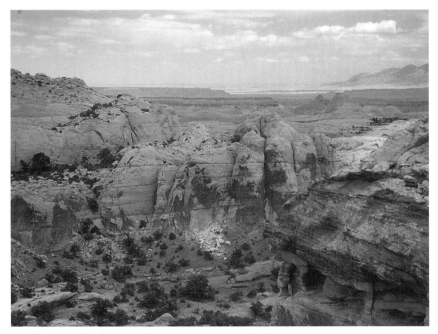

Waterpocket Fold and Henry Mountains from Navajo Knobs

traditional stopping point for cattlemen driving their herds through the Waterpocket Fold country.

Description

Peek-a-boo Rock can be viewed in the northwest from the trailhead, and the menacing saw-toothed profile of Waterpocket Fold fills the horizon from the northwest to the southeast, rearing its majestic slickrock skyward. We begin our jaunt (4900') by following the trail along the left side of a fence. This leads across greasewood-clad flats generally westward toward a low sandstone knoll. The trail drops into the wash where we turn right and slog through the sand amid red slabs of Carmel Formation rocks. Soon the fence reappears above us and east of the wash, which presently bends west, cutting deeply into towering slickrock.

Before long we enter a narrow slot barely 2–3 feet wide, with sheer walls rising nearly 300 feet above on either side. Beyond the confines of these narrows, Gambel oak and boxelder appear. Ahead we bushwhack through dense vegetation, scramble over or around boulders, and slog through deep sand, but despite these obstacles this mysterious canyon lures us onward.

Eventually the wash abruptly ends below a moderately steep slickrock chute at 1.5 miles (5420'). At this point we should turn around and return the way we came. ■

Hike 25. Halls Creek Overlook to Brimhall Bridge

Distance	4.6 miles round trip
Elevation gain	1050'
Average hiking time	4 hours
Difficulty	5
Child rating	3
Best seasons	April through mid-June; mid-September through November
Hazards	Steep scrambling over slickrock and talus; possible quicksand; deep wading and possibly a brief swim of a deep pothole; flash-flood danger.

Driving to the trailhead

Follow driving directions for Hike 23 to reach the junction of the Burr Trail and Notom-Bullfrog roads, and proceed southeast on the Notom-Bullfrog Road for 10.9 miles to a prominently signed 3-way junction, where you turn right onto the paved road, heading towards HALLS CREEK OVER-LOOK-4 and BULLFROG BASIN-25. The road ahead follows a shallow valley toward the south, reaching a junction after 1 mile with a southwest-bound dirt road signed for HALLS CREEK OVERLOOK and TRAILHEAD.

Turn right and follow the rough dirt road west-southwest along a draw south of a minor wash, then climb a broken sandstone slope, soon topping out on the gentle terrain of Big Thomson Mesa. (Note: avoid this dirt road during and shortly after rainfall, when its clay surface becomes impassable.) The road ahead is still rough, and shortly you reach a third and final junction after 2.5 miles, also signed for the overlook. Turn right once again, and follow the very rocky and rough dirt road, passable only to high-clearance or 4WD vehicles. A single pullout at this point affords parking for a passenger car. The road ends at a small turnaround and picnic area at Halls Creek Overlook, 2.8 miles from the paved road.

Introduction

A strenuous and demanding dayhike recommended only for experienced desert hikers, this short but memorable trip offers rewards commensurate with the effort it requires. The trail descends steeply from the rim of Big Thomson Mesa into the valley of Halls Creek, then ascends a precipitous defile to an overlook of the bridge. This canyon is passable only by the experienced desert hiker. There is no shade except within the confines of Brimhall Canyon, and this part of the park is extremely hot in summer.

Before beginning the hike, pause to soak in the vistas from the trailhead. Halls Creek Overlook lies at the west rim of the broad, grass- and shrub-clad expanse of Big Thomson Mesa. Magnificent vistas reach eastward beyond distant, higher mesas to the Little Rockies, and northeast to the higher prominences of the Henry Mountains. Colorful shale slopes drape the lower flanks of the Henrys from Mt. Hillers northward, but the sedimentary strata abruptly give way to the igneous rocks that compose Henry Mountains.

We can see a 40-mile stretch of the Waterpocket Fold, rising above the narrow valley of Halls Creek, from the northwest near The Post to near its southern terminus above presently invisible Lake Powell in the southeast. Notice how the fold becomes progressively lower toward the south. Gazing northwest along the fold, we can plainly see how steeply the rock strata have been tilted, especially where the Kayenta rocks, featuring distinct layering, overlie the white Navajo Sandstone—the dominant rock of the fold. In places we can also see part of the Circle Cliffs, which bound the western flanks of the fold, and far to the southeast are heat-hazy buttes rising beyond the Colorado River near Glen Canyon Dam and Page, Arizona.

Description

From the trailhead (5278'), our rough, rocky trail descends northwest along the cliff face of Big Thomson Mesa, passing through a variety of rock strata: the Dakota Sandstone that caps the rim; the Brushy Basin Shale forming the bench below; the Salt Wash Sandstone forming the rim of the bench; the Summerville Formation; and finally the Entrada Sandstone. But all these strata are largely obscured by conglomeratic boulders fallen from the rim, and are difficult to discern one from another. Enroute, we enjoy expansive vistas of the Waterpocket Fold and Halls Creek, with the redrock prominence of Deer Point, in the west-southwest, and other crags atop the Circle Cliffs rising above.

After negotiating several steep, rocky switchbacks, we emerge onto a slope clad in blackbrush and more boulders, and cross a low ridge between domes of red Entrada Sandstone pitted with solution cavities. Beyond, our well-defined trail heads across a shrubby bench, soon reaching a sign along cottonwood-lined Halls Creek wash at 1.2 miles (4460'). The sign lists several destinations and mileages, but from here on the routes are not well-marked.

To reach the mouth of Brimhall Canyon, cross the wash and follow the trail southwest along a bench decorated with grasses, sagebrush, rabbitbrush, juniper, and scattered and picturesque, excessively branched cottonwoods.

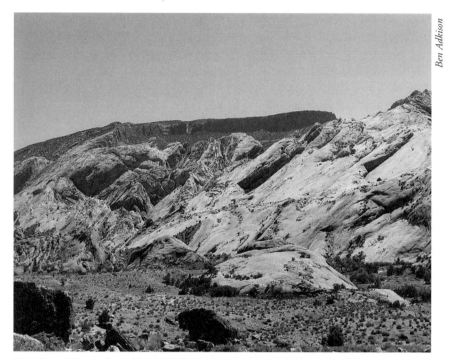

Ben Adkison

Deer Point, Waterpocket Fold, and Halls Creek valley from Halls Creek Overlook

Brimhall Canyon is the first drainage on our right, 0.2 mile from the sign. Vegetation abruptly changes as we enter the canyon, noticing a grove of Gambel oak growing at the base of a steep slickrock slope of Navajo Sandstone. Here runoff from Brimhall Canyon saturates the ground, providing ample moisture for the oaks. The slickrock above absorbs very little water, and its runoff provides more moisture. This dampness, combined with the shade and shelter the steep slickrock slope provides, creates a microclimate. Abundant vegetation, some of which grows to atypical proportions due to the canyon microclimate, clothes the lower canyon.

Pause at the canyon's mouth to gaze up into its spectacular labyrinth, where tall cliffs of Navajo Sandstone frame the ledgy, broken slopes of the Kayenta Formation and the massive steep slopes of orange-hued Wingate Sandstone beyond, sliced by numerous shallow gullies.

After 0.25 mile the canyon appears to end in a boulder-choked chute below a tall, dry waterfall, but actually the main canyon makes a 90° bend toward the north here. At this point we must briefly climb the slickrock to our right to continue. Ahead we traverse more slickrock above a narrow chute, then proceed along the boulder-littered wash. Soon the canyon bends sharply west, becoming very narrow, and we are quickly confronted by yet another obstacle, a deep pool. This pool requires a deep wade, or more likely a brief swim, to continue up the canyon. Exiting the pool, we must climb over the large boulders that choke these narrows.

Ahead, more boulders choke the canyon, further impeding progress. But 0.6 mile up the canyon we reach another deep pool, lying beneath a 12-foot waterfall. From here, we scramble up the slope rising above to the right, northwest, taking care among the loose boulders and sand.

Our ascent ends atop a minor ridge at 2.1 miles (4780'), where we enjoy a head-on view of Brimhall Bridge, lying directly west across the canyon. Brimhall Bridge boasts two spans, both arcing over a deep alcove. A shallow gully has developed on the hummocky Wingate slope, its runoff pouring under the bridges and helping to enlarge them. Another alcove has developed high above the canyon near Brimhall Bridge, and it will perhaps evolve into another bridge that may attract visitors in the distant future, perhaps long after Brimhall Bridge has been reduced to rubble by the inexorable forces of erosion.

From our vantage we notice how the massive domes and walls of the Navajo abruptly give way to the softer, broken rocks of the Kayenta, which in turn give way to the hummocky slickrock slopes of the Wingate, upon which the bridge has formed. To get a closer look at the bridge, we can work our way briefly northwest along this ridge, cross a narrow, minor canyon, and carefully descend ledges of Kayenta rocks for another 0.2 mile to the canyon bottom opposite the bridge (4700').

Return the way you came. ■

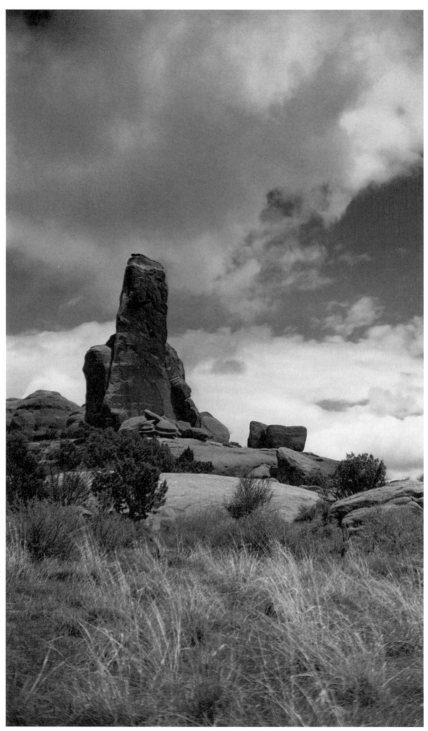

Dark Angel, Devils Garden

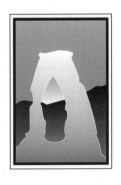

Arches
National Park

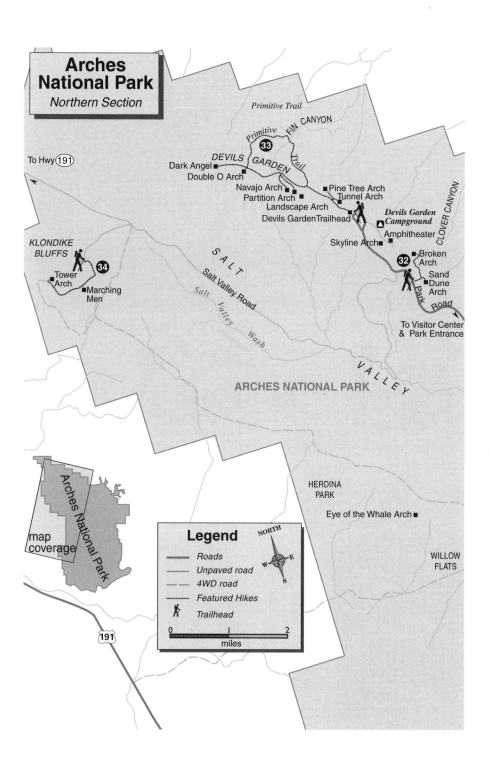

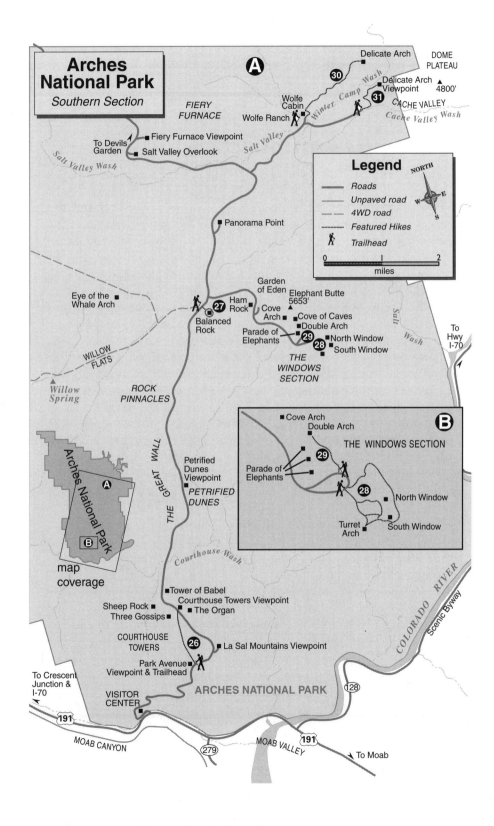

Arches National Park
Southern Section

FIERY FURNACE

Delicate Arch ■

DOME PLATEAU

30

Delicate Arch
Viewpoint
31

▲ 4800'

CACHE VALLEY

Cache Valley Wash

Wolfe Cabin
Wolfe Ranch

Winter Camp Wash

■ Fiery Furnace Viewpoint
■ Salt Valley Overlook

To Devils Garden

Salt Valley Wash

Salt Valley Wash

Salt Valley

■ Panorama Point

Legend

NORTH

Roads
Unpaved road
4WD road
Featured Hikes
Trailhead

0   1   2
miles

W N E
S

Eye of the
Whale Arch ■

Garden of Eden
Ham Rock ■   Elephant Butte
27   5653' ▲
Cove
Balanced   Arch ■   Cove of Caves
Rock   ■ Double Arch
Parade of   29   ■ North Window
Elephants   28   ■ South Window

THE WINDOWS SECTION

Salt Wash

To Hwy I-70

WILLOW FLATS

▲ Willow Spring

ROCK PINNACLES

THE GREAT WALL

Petrified Dunes Viewpoint
PETRIFIED DUNES

B   THE WINDOWS SECTION

■ Cove Arch
Double Arch

29

Parade of
Elephants

28   ■ North Window

Turret
Arch ■   ■ South Window

Courthouse Wash

Arches National Park

A

B

map coverage

COLORADO RIVER

Scenic Byway

■ Tower of Babel
Courthouse Towers Viewpoint
Sheep Rock ■   ■ The Organ
Three Gossips ■

COURTHOUSE TOWERS

26   ■ La Sal Mountains Viewpoint

Park Avenue
Viewpoint & Trailhead

ARCHES NATIONAL PARK

128

To Crescent
Junction & I-70

VISITOR CENTER

191

MOAB CANYON

279

MOAB VALLEY

191

To Moab

Introduction

Arches National Park encompasses 76,519 acres of desert and slickrock in east-central Utah, and is one of the most delightful national parks on the Colorado Plateau. The park is small enough that many of its primary features can be viewed from the road, yet large enough to provide a rewarding backcountry experience for adventurous dayhikers. The unique examples of nature's and architecture are not on a grand scale here, but nevertheless the landscapes in the park evoke awe and wonder in anyone who gazes upon them.

Arches are natural stone openings found throughout the sandstone formations on the Colorado Plateau, but are quite rare elsewhere in the world. They can be found in virtually every national park in Utah, but in Arches National Park there is a profusion of these openings; nowhere else on the globe does the concentration of arches approach that within this small park.

One of the most common questions asked by park visitors is: how many arches are there in the park? The answer depends on the definition of an arch. Openings in Arches National Park vary in size from fist-sized holes to those that span hundreds of feet, but for practical purposes an arch is defined as an aperture that has a "light opening" of at least 3 feet. The opening can be 3 feet by 1 foot, 3 feet by 3 feet, 3 feet by 50 feet, etc. Using this criterion, there were more than 2000 known such openings within the park as of 1991.

However, natural arches are only a small part of the overall scene in the park. Pinnacles, towers, cliffs, deep canyons, broad grassy valleys, and a rainbow of colorful rocks foreground distant views of endless deserts, lofty alpine peaks, wooded mesas, and vast plateaus.

Arches National Park lies on a gently sloping highland, the Salt Valley Anticline. It rises gently from the desert valleys that flank its west, north, and east sides; along its south edge, the the highland rises abruptly, due to past movement along the Moab Fault. The crest of the gently rising bulge in the earth has long since collapsed and eroded away, forming a trough that bisects the park, separating two parallel ridges that host the salmon-tinted fins of rock in which arches have formed. The south part of the park is more complex, consisting of a profusion of monoliths, towers, brush-clad flats, extensive areas of hummocky slickrock, and two deep, serpentine canyons—Courthouse Wash and Salt Wash.

The fascinating landscape of Arches beckons hikers to explore its secrets. When you visit, park your car and walk the trails or explore the untracked reaches of the backcountry. This land is magical, its images are powerful, and your memories will last a lifetime.

Plants and animals of Arches

The casual observer at Arches sees a landscape dominated by rock and sand, with a few coarse shrubs here and a scattering of gnarled, stunted trees there. But a closer look reveals a wide variety of trees, shrubs, and wildflowers inhabiting every space where soil has collected.

The most obvious and abundant plant community in the park is the pinyon-juniper woodland. This pygmy forest of small, drab, gnarled, and weather-tortured trees covers nearly half the park. It is not true forest, however; the trees tend to be scattered discontinuously throughout their range. Utah juniper, typically squat and multibranched, dominates in this zone. Two-needled or Colorado pinyon (also called nut pine since it often produces a crop of tasty nuts) grows with juniper at higher elevations, where there is a slight increase in precipitation and temperatures are somewhat cooler. Pinyons also like the sheltered environment of cliff bases, where runoff from the slickrock above provides moisture. Shrubs growing among these gnarled trees include cliffrose, singleleaf ash, squawbush, wavyleaf oak, littleleaf mountain mahogany, Fremont barberry, Utah serviceberry, and blackbrush, which occasionally creeps into the pinyon-juniper woodland

The desert-shrub plant community is the second most common in the park, occupying sand dunes, sand and clay slopes, and flats. From a distance, these low shrubs lend a dull gray appearance to the landscape. Blackbrush is the dominant shrub in this community, but in areas of high alkalinity it is replaced by salt-tolerant shrubs, such as greasewood—a spiny shrub with fleshy leaves. Four-wing saltbush, mat saltbush, shadscale, and pickleweed also grow on alkaline soils, whereas sand sagebrush and the aromatic purple sage prefer sandier areas within the broad range of this plant community.

The riparian woodland differs from other plant communities in the park in that its inhabitants require abundant and constant moisture. Salt Wash and Courthouse Wash both have fine examples of this woodland. Even if the wash appears dry, considerable underground moisture resides wherever these plants grow. Fremont cottonwood, coyote and sandbar willow, and tamarisk are abundant in riparian woodlands. These green ribbons of vegetation stand in marked contrast to the sparse shrublands and slickrock that surround them.

In spring, the fresh green prairies of the grasslands plant community contrast with drab shrublands and colorful cliffs and fins. Grasslands are dominated by a multitude of grasses, including sand dropseed, Indian ricegrass, galleta, and purple three-awn, plus many more that only the trained eye of a botanist would discern. Although grasslands are almost devoid of shrubs, winter fat—a low native shrub with small, white-woolly leaves— grows in the park's grasslands, and is important as winter browse for the area's mule deer. Overgrazing by domestic stock animals has led to the introduction of non-native plant species in Salt Valley's grasslands. Brome, or cheatgrass, is a particular nuisance to hikers because its pointed seeds work their way into socks and irritate one's legs.

Hanging gardens are a beautiful and delicate plant community in Arches, whose inhabitants require a constant source of moisture. They typically occur in sheltered alcoves or on shady canyon walls where water seeps from the sandstone, most often along a horizontal fracture or just above an impermeable layer of rock. These hanging gardens contrast vividly with the harsh landscape of naked stone upon which they thrive. Maidenhair fern, scarlet monkey flower, alcove columbine, poison ivy, and giant helleborine orchid are among hanging gardens' lush, water-loving plants.

Like desert plants, animals have also adapted to the rigors of the high desert environment. Many are nocturnal, avoiding the heat of the day by venturing from their homes at night to seek food and water. Exceedingly high surface temperatures during summer drive these animals to tuck themselves away in cool burrows. Some live close to water sources or hibernate in anticipation of the next major rainfall. The Ord's kangaroo rat is a seldom-seen nocturnal animal. It is noteworthy because it rarely drinks water, but instead obtains moisture internally through the metabolism of seeds.

Birds are the most abundant and noticeable creatures in the park, and are most active during morning and late afternoon hours. Some birds are residents, while others are migratory, visiting the park seasonally. White-throated swifts, violet-green swallows, and canyon wrens flit among canyon cliffs. The song sparrow, common flicker, blue grosbeak are some of the great variety of birds that traverse the park's watercourses. The spotted sandpiper, warbling vireo, house wren, common raven, and Bullock's oriole are others that frequent the park's rivers and streams, where an abundant supply of insects makes for a constant food source.

Raptors such as the red-tailed hawk, kestrel, and prairie falcon soar above Arches' grasslands. Nighthawks swiftly carve circles, dive, and soar in pursuit of insects in the morning and evening hours; their distinctive song is unmistakable. Other birds of the grasslands include the western meadowlark, mourning dove, common raven, and horned lark. Sparrows and finches are common denizens of the park's scrublands. Pinyon-juniper woodlands host pinyon and scrub jays, house finches, ash-throated flycatchers, gray vireos, black-throated gray warblers, plain titmouses, and various woodpeckers. Arches is home to many more birds, particularly in spring, when food is most abundant. Their melodious songs and flashes of color are important parts of the Arches experience.

Of all the animals in Arches, lizards are second only to birds among those most commonly observed. The northern plateau lizard, leopard lizard, western whiptail, desert spiny lizard, short-horned lizard, collared lizard, and sagebrush lizard are the most common ones. Only one poisonous snake is found in Arches, the midget faded rattlesnake. Native to the Colorado Plateau of Colorado and eastern Utah, it is not particularly common in Arches. It averages only about 18 inches in length, and is typically straw-colored. Like other rattlesnakes, it is not particularly aggressive, and would rather be left alone by human visitors. All other snakes in the park are harmless, including the gopher snake, Mesa Verde night snake, and the racer snake. These, as well as the common, black-necked, and wandering garter snakes are typically found near water.

Numerous mammals live in Arches. The mule deer is the park's largest and perhaps most common mammal, but to catch a glimpse of it, you will probably have to explore off of established trails or hike in the morning or evening hours. Bighorn sheep might reveal themselves in the southwest part of the park near The Great Wall west of The Windows. These secretive creatures were rarely sighted in the park before 1985, when park officials transplanted 30 sheep from Canyonlands National Park in an attempt to reestablish a herd in Arches, part of its former range.

Other mammals include coyotes, whose eerie howls in the evening and at night attests to their presence, although these reticent canines are not readily observed. Among their prey is the desert cottontail, commonly seen darting from bush to bush seeking protection from predators such as coyotes and hawks. The long ears of blacktail jackrabbits and desert cottontails serve as "radiators" to dissipate body heat. Other park animals visitors might encounter include the rock squirrel, whitetail antelope squirrel, and bats such as the western pipistrel.

In a land of parched, naked stone, it is difficult to imagine the existence of frogs and toads, but six species of these amphibians make their homes in Arches. They are found only in moist areas along Courthouse Wash, the Colorado River, Salt Wash, and intermittent streams and ephemeral potholes.

Interpretive activities

Arches has a wide variety of things to see and do, whether you stay only half a day or several days. To make the most of your trip, stop at the visitor center, located just beyond the park entrance station. Books, maps, an interpretive museum, slide shows, and a knowledgeable staff are available to answer any questions one may have about the park or the surrounding area.

The visitor center operates with extended hours from mid-March through mid-October, and 8 A.M.–4:30 P.M. in winter.

Interpretive activities in the park include evening amphitheater programs in the Devils Garden Campground each night from spring through fall. Ranger-led walks follow a variety of short trails. The Fiery Furnace hike is a favorite of park visitors, and guided hikes are conducted there twice daily. Make advance reservations and purchase tickets for this popular hike at the visitor center. A schedule of interpretive activities is posted at the visitor center and at the campground.

Most interpretive activities, however, are directed toward self-guiding trails, and an excellent guide entitled "A Road Guide to Arches National Park" allows visitors to get the most from their drive through Arches. Self-guided trails include the Devils Garden Trail, the 0.2-mile Desert Nature Trail, and trails in the Wolfe Ranch Historic District. Trail guides are available at trailheads and at the visitor center.

Campgrounds

The 52-site Devils Garden Campground is the only vehicle camping area in the park. This is one of the most scenic and delightful campgrounds in all of Utah's national parks. The campsites are situated along a 0.75-mile-long road in the southern reaches of Devils Garden, encircled by slickrock fins and shaded by scattered pinyons and junipers. Various shrubs and wildflowers decorate this natural rock garden, and the campground's location on a highland offers tremendous panoramas across endless desert and mesas that stretch eastward into Colorado. A campground fee is charged, and campers are limited to 14 days. Campers must register for the campground at the visitor center or at the park entrance station.

Three picnic areas are widely scattered throughout Arches. The first lies deep in Moab Canyon next to the visitor center. The second, opposite Balanced Rock, has little shade but features far-ranging panoramas stretching as far away as the lofty La Sal Mountains. The third picnic area lies in the incomparable Devils Garden area, nestled against sheer slickrock fins just short of the campground entrance.

Moab, only 5 miles from Arches, is a small but bustling community that is the hub of recreational activity in the canyon country of eastern Utah. Moab offers a full line of services to meet the needs of most any visitor to Canyon Country. Groceries, gas, and limited backpacking supplies are available here, as well as 16 private campgrounds, 30 motels, 17 bed and breakfasts, and 51 guest houses, apartment accommodations, condos and cabins. Those who prefer a guided tour of Canyon Country have numerous outfitters from which to choose. Tours range from float trips on the Colorado and Green rivers to jeep trips on any number of 4WD roads in the area.

Camping in the area ranges from spacious private campgrounds around Moab to primitive camping on Bureau of Land Management lands. Many visitors camp alongside the Colorado River upstream from the Moab Bridge along Utah Highway 128; since this area has been overused, camping is now restricted to designated sites. Other primitive sites can be found throughout the area on Bureau of Land Management lands. Two Forest Service campgrounds located alongside lakes high in the La Sal Mountains offer a pleasant refuge from the searing heat of summer.

For more information on the park, lodging, guide services, and campgrounds, contact:

Park Superintendent
Arches National Park
P.O. Box 907
Moab, UT 84532
(435) 259-8161

Moab Information Center
Center and Main streets
Moab, UT 84532

U.S. Forest Service
Manti-La Sal National Forest
2290 South West Resource Blvd.
Moab, UT 84532
(435) 259-7155

Hiking in Arches

Arches has such a wide variety of trails that it may be difficult to choose among them. Ranging in length from 0.1 mile to the 7-mile Devils Garden trail system, most trails have arches as their primary destination. Other trails traverse canyons, slickrock, and grassy desert parks. With more than a dozen developed routes—many that lead to destinations only a few minutes walk from the trailhead—Arches has something for hikers of all abilities.

Most of the developed trails in Arches are fairly short and present no major difficulties for novice hikers. The Delicate Arch Trail and the primitive part of the Devils Garden Trail are exceptions and should be avoided by acrophobic visitors. Many trails have cairned sections across slickrock, which can be slippery when wet. Hiking in the canyons is largely restricted to wash bottoms, but in open country hikers are limited only by their ability and the extent of their desire to discover the secrets of the desert.

Arches National Park can be enjoyed year-round, but spring and fall usually offer the most comfortable weather. To learn more about hiking seasons, refer to the section "Hiking Utah's desert parks", in the introduction. Bugs, flash floods, and extreme heat are some of the hazards hikers may encounter in Arches.

There are no dependable water sources in Arches. The only perennial stream, Salt Wash, is too brackish and fouled by cattle to be potable. No day-hiker should enter the backcountry without ample water. ■

Hike 26. Park Avenue

Distance	0.9 mile shuttle trip
Elevation loss	320'
Average hiking time	30 minutes
Difficulty rating	2
Child rating	2
Best seasons	April through mid-June; mid-September through November
Hazards	Negligible

Driving to the trailhead

Arches National Park can be reached by driving 26 miles southeast on U.S. 191 from Crescent Junction on Interstate 70, located 20 miles east of Green River, Utah. The signed turnoff to the park also lies 5 miles northwest of Moab, and 2 miles from the Colorado River bridge on U.S. 191.

From the turnoff in the depths of cliffbound Moab Canyon, the park road quickly descends to the park entrance station. Entrance fees must be paid to enter the park. A park map and information about campsites are available here.

Just beyond the entrance station lies the park visitor center. From there, the park road curves upward beneath tall cliffs. After 2.2 miles from U.S. 191 you reach the signed Park Avenue turnout along the north side of the road, where the Park Avenue Trail begins.

To locate the terminus of the trail, follow the park road for 1.2 miles beyond the Park Avenue parking area to the Courthouse Towers Viewpoint parking area.

Introduction

The Park Avenue Trail, an easy downhill stroll in a high desert canyon, leads the hiker among towering slickrock cliffs and stony battlements, nature's counterpart to a city street among lofty skyscrapers. This trip offers a fine introduction to the great monoliths of the Courthouse Towers, plus views of long-ruined arches and of one of the youngest arches visible from any trail in the park. Hikers who can't manage the car shuttle should consider taking the trail as a round trip, or hike part way through Park Avenue from either trailhead.

Description

From the trailhead (4560') with a splendid view of the La Sal Mountains behind and the cliffs of the Courthouse Towers ahead, follow the paved path that leads 100 yards to the Park Avenue Viewpoint. This point offers an awe-inspiring view into the heart of the Courthouse Towers, where near-vertical redrock fins and towers dominate the scene.

Most park visitors go no farther, but for a more intimate perspective, bear left just before the viewpoint and follow the dirt trail into the wash below (Park Avenue). Flanked on either side by towering fins (the fins to your right—northeast—are perhaps the eroded remnants of two prehistoric arches), follow the wash downhill among a scattering of twisted Utah juniper, blackbrush, Mormon Tea, wavyleaf oak, singleleaf ash, and cliffrose. True to its name, this route is reminiscent of walking among skyscrapers on a city street. The cliffs and fins of Courthouse Towers, composed of the Slick Rock member, stand upon the thin layer of the comparatively softer, contorted Dewey Bridge member of the Entrada Sandstone.

Soon the floor of our wash-bottom route is dominated by the whitish slickrock of the Navajo Sandstone. Ahead on the northern horizon looms the giant monolith of the Tower of Babel. At 4537 feet elevation, this impressive tower soars nearly 300 feet above its surroundings.

As we approach the park road near the end of our scenic jaunt, notice a large pinnacle at the north end of the fin on the left (west). Most likely this pinnacle was once the north abutment of an ancient arch, long since collapsed. Such erosional remnants of arches are seen in many places in the park, but are particularly abundant in the Courthouse Towers region. Here you'll see boulders littering the gap between the pinnacle and the main fin, further evidence that an arch once stood there.

The Three Gossips, a group of three imposing, boulder-capped pinnacles, soon rise above us to the northwest. Finally, at an arrow sign under the shadow of the 250-foot spire of The Organ, we leave the potholed slickrock of the wash and quickly climb to the park road opposite the Courthouse Towers Viewpoint to end the hike after 0.9 mile.

From the viewpoint at this trailhead, aptly named and isolated Sheep Rock rises to the northwest, separated from the main fin by a rather large void. This is perhaps the finest example of a collapsed arch in the park. Sheep Rock formed the north abutment of what must have been a huge arch. A tiny arch, known as Hole-in-the-Wall or Baby Arch, has penetrated the wall of the main fin to the left of the void. The angular outline of this opening and the boulders littering its base, not yet removed by the forces of erosion, attest to its youth. ■

Hike 27. Balanced Rock Trail

Distance	0.3 mile semiloop trip
Elevation gain	25'
Average hiking time	20 minutes
Difficulty rating	1
Child rating	1
Best season	All year
Hazards	Negligible

Driving to the trailhead

Follow driving directions for Hike 26 to reach Arches National Park, then follow the paved park road generally north for 8.7 miles to the signed Balanced Rock parking area on the east side of the road. This parking area lies 0.2 mile south of The Windows spur road.

Introduction

Three redrock monoliths jut above a gentle highland, guarding the approach to the scenic Windows Section of the park. The most famous and distinctive of these pinnacles is Balanced Rock. The rock seems to defy gravity as it rises 55 feet above a pedestal that itself rises 73 feet above ground level. Composed of the erosion-resistant Slick Rock member of the Entrada Sandstone, Balanced Rock protects the softer pedestal, composed of the Entrada's Dewey Bridge member.

This pleasant stroll not only offers a close-up view of Balanced Rock, but also yields far-reaching vistas of distant mountains, colorful cliffs, and wooded mesas. Balanced Rock and all arches named on the USGS topographic maps are closed to rock climbing.

Description

This trail crests a hill between a monolith fin to the north (Bubo) and imposing Balanced Rock directly above to the south. Its huge boulder appears much larger from beneath than it does from the trailhead. The whitish rock this pinnacle rests upon is the Navajo Sandstone, well exposed across the plateau to the south and southeast. Scattered redrock pinnacles resting atop the Navajo punctuate the landscape and foreground impressive vistas of the La Sal Mountains, a cluster of 12,000-foot summits on the southeast horizon.

Other notable views include massive Elephant Butte toward the east-southeast, accentuated by the fascinating Parade of Elephants and the openings of Turret Arch and Double Arch, 2 miles distant.

After descending below the east side of Balanced Rock, the route bends west and climbs to a minor gap between that rock and the third of this impressive triad of pinnacles, to the south. We then descend easily northwest to rejoin the access trail, then quickly backtrack to the trailhead. ■

Hike 28. North Window, Turret Arch, and South Window Trails

Distance	Up to 1.1 miles round trip or loop trip
Elevation gain	140'
Average hiking time	About 1 hour
Difficulty rating	1
Child rating	1 to 2
Best seasons	April through mid-June; mid-September through November
Hazards	Negligible

Driving to the trailhead

Follow driving directions for Hike 26 to reach Arches National Park, then follow the paved park road generally north for 8.9 miles to the eastbound spur road signed for The Windows Section. Follow that paved road for 2.6 miles to the parking area in the loop at the road's end.

Introduction

A network of short but very scenic trails begins at the roadend in The Windows Section of the park. These popular trails can be arranged into a variety of interesting loop hikes that visit some of the best-known and easily accessible arches in the park. More experienced hikers may wish to loop back to the trailhead from South Window via the so-called primitive trail, leaving the crowds behind and enjoying broad panoramas. Due to the large numbers of visitors who follow these trails every year, the park requires that visitors stay on the trails to alleviate resource damage.

Description

From the trailhead (5160'), the wide trail to The Windows leads southeast across a blackbrush-dotted flat for 0.1 mile and then forks. The right fork continues southeast, climbing gently for another 0.1 mile to a junction. The right-branching trail from this junction quickly leads to Turret Arch, while the left-branching trail leads to North Window. The North and South windows are visible along either route.

If you take the short right-branching trail to Turret Arch, you'll see that, unlike many arches in the park, Turret Arch's opening is taller than it is wide, 64 feet high versus 39 feet wide. Two smaller openings penetrate this large, isolated hogback fin. The larger is 12 feet wide by 13 feet high; the smaller is only 8 feet high by 4.5 feet wide.

This trail then heads northeast for less than 0.1 mile, where it meets the previous junction's left-branching trail between the North and South Windows. From this junction, the left-fork trail leads back north to North Window, while the right-fork trail heads east to South Window.

Back at the junction 0.1 mile from the parking area, if you branch east onto the left-fork trail, instead of visiting Turret Arch, you'll follow this rock-lined trail easily up over Navajo Sandstone slickrock. Just north of North Window is an arch-like alcove. On the opposite side of the alcove, as viewed from the primitive trail, yet another alcove has formed. This is a good example of the way many arches in the park form. As erosion continues, an even larger opening will form. Hence this alcove has been dubbed "Arch-in-the-Making."

After 0.25 mile from the start of the left-fork trail, we reach the opening of North Window. This opening is at the contact point of two members of the Entrada Sandstone: the lower half of the abutments of North Window is made up of the basal unit of the Entrada, the Dewey Bridge member. The overlying and consequently younger Slick Rock member forms the top of the arch as well as the crest of the large fin through which the arch has penetrated. This is an excellent spot in which to observe the nature of the comparatively soft Dewey Bridge member, which forms the base of most arches in the park and features a contorted, blocky, and irregular surface. The Slick Rock member, in contrast, is quite smooth and often exhibits sheer, unjointed cliffs. As the softer Dewey Bridge member erodes, the openings often enlarge.

Large North Window (51 feet high by 93 feet wide) frames exceptional vistas, reaching east across miles of great redrock mesas and cliffs bounding the invisible gorge of the Colorado River.

The trail proceeds south for about 150 yards to a junction with the right-fork and Turret Arch trails. This junction lies below a large, nose-like protrusion between North and South windows. The right-fork trail leads to Turret Arch; we follow the left-fork trail, bound for South Window.

After briefly leading south, the left-fork trail rounds the nose-like fin and quickly reaches the expansive opening of South Window, which penetrates the redrock fin farther above ground than its northern counterpart does.

An interesting trail looping back to the parking area east of The Windows begins at South Window. Designated a primitive trail, the route is nevertheless easy to follow, though its tread is not as excessively wide and graded as the primary Windows trails. It offers expansive vistas and a brief opportunity to escape the throngs of tourists pounding out the main trails in The Windows Section.

From the foot of South Window, cairns lead the way along a small, east-trending wash. The trail becomes more apparent as it quickly arcs to the north, and both windows soon come into view as we traverse below and east of them.

Wallflower is a common springtime blossom here, a cluster of yellow flowers borne on a single stalk. It grows among pinyons, junipers, black-brush, Mormon Tea, wavyleaf oak, singleleaf ash, yucca, and prickly pear, which boasts its own vivid blooms in late spring.

Soon the trail crosses the slickrock opposite a large, tunnel-like alcove. Weathering and gravity will, in the not-too-distant future, cause this alcove and another on the opposite side of the fin to merge, adding another arch to the catalog of openings in the park. Our easy-to-follow trail descends slightly, and we can gaze east beyond the almost imperceptible gash of Salt Wash's lower canyon to broad Dry Mesa, laced by several mineral exploration roads 3 miles to the east.

A short stretch across slickrock ensues, bringing us to a gap in the fin between two interesting pinnacles. From the gap, our trail descends quickly west into the broad head of a wash. After reaching the brushy flats below, the trail meanders southwest to the nearby trailhead to complete this pleasant, scenic, albeit short, loop, 0.6 mile from South Window. ■

Hike 29. Double Arch Trail

Distance	0.4 mile round trip
Elevation gain	80'
Average hiking time	20 to 30 minutes
Difficulty rating	1
Child rating	1
Best seasons	April through mid-June; mid-September through November
Hazards	Negligible

Driving to the trailhead

Follow driving directions for Hike 26 to reach Arches National Park, then follow the paved park road generally north for 8.9 miles to the eastbound spur road signed for The Windows Section. Follow that paved road for 2.6 miles to the loop at the road's end, then curve back the way you came for 0.2 mile to the Double Arch parking area on the north side of the road.

Introduction

This easy and highly scenic stroll is suitable for hikers of every ability. Double Arch, above the trail's end, is the second largest natural rock opening in the park. Its eastern arch spans 160 feet between abutments and rises 105 feet above the ground. The smaller western arch opens into the Cove of Caves, and is 60 feet wide and 61 feet high.

Description

From the signed trailhead at 5150 feet, the wide trail undulates over a corrugated flat, dotted with scattered junipers and the ubiquitous blackbrush. Double Arch lies ahead to the northwest, just to the left of a keyhole-shaped alcove suspended high on the wall above the flats. Nearby lies a larger, similarly shaped alcove known as Archaeological Cave.

The trail passes the east side of Parade of Elephants, and ends beneath the larger, easternmost span of Double Arch at 0.2 mile (5200'). This is one of the most interesting arches in the park, and it actually boasts three openings if you consider the opening on top between the two arches. The top, or third, opening may be a pothole-type arch, and the formation of the pothole and the consequent concentration and seepage of groundwater probably led to the formation of alcoves and ultimately Double Arch.

From Double Arch, return the way you came. ■

Hike 30. Delicate Arch Trail

Distance	3.0 miles round trip
Elevation gain	560'
Average hiking time	1½ to 2 hours
Difficulty rating	3
Child rating	3
Best seasons	April through mid-June; mid-September through November
Hazards	No shade; steep dropoffs

Driving to the trailhead

Follow driving directions for Hike 26 to reach Arches National Park, then follow the paved park road generally north for 11.2 miles to the junction with the spur road to Wolfe Ranch, Delicate Arch Trailhead, and Delicate Arch Viewpoint.

Turn right onto the spur road and drive 1.2 miles to another short spur road leading quickly north to the parking area at Wolfe Ranch.

Introduction

Park visitors with time enough to hike only one or two short trails should put the trail to Delicate Arch at the top of their itineraries. This trip is arguably the most scenic of all the hikes in the park; it climbs slickrock slopes, passes hanging gardens thriving in hidden alcoves, and ends at a dramatic overlook of the park's most famous rock span, a lone, arching ribbon of stone aptly named Delicate Arch.

Superb vistas range from vast expanses of slickrock to wooded mesas and sheer cliffs and the lofty La Sal Mountains, which form an impressive backdrop of alpine peaks approaching 13,000 feet in elevation.

At the end of the trip is a narrow catwalk of trail, carved into the face of a sheer cliff. Acrophobic hikers might instead consider the shorter trail to Delicate Arch Viewpoint (Hike 31) for a fine, but more distant, view of this isolated span of stone.

Description

This popular trail begins at the site of Wolfe Ranch (4280'), the only homestead ever established in what is now Arches National Park. Beyond a cabin our trail crosses (via a sturdy steel bridge) the perennial, alkaline stream draining Salt Wash. It first heads across a greasewood-clad flat, then climbs onto the coarse Salt Wash Sandstone member of the Morrison Formation.

A short spur trail to a Ute Indian petroglyph panel branches to the left, just before a switchback. We don't want to miss this site, one of only two easily accessible rock-writing sites in the park. This fine panel depicts riders on horseback, bighorn sheep (an important food source to native peoples), and what appear to be two dogs. It is believed to be of relatively recent origin, since horses were not introduced to the area's Ute people until the early 1700s.

Presently, a view of South Window captures our attention to the south across Cache Valley. A towering wall of Wingate Sandstone flanks each side of the portal of lower Salt Wash, viewed across the valley to the south.

Beyond a bench our smooth, rock-lined trail soon drops into the jumbled topography of an east-west fault zone. As the trail begins to rise through this corrugated landscape, we soon pass into the red shales of the Tidwell member of the Morrison Formation, where slopes are punctuated by numerous large siliceous outcroppings. As we climb a red-colored hill and leave the corrugated basin, we can glimpse a seep-fed hanging garden in a split-level alcove in the wall to our north, resplendent with verdant growth.

Cairns lead our way over the slickrock of the Moab Tongue, and steps cut into the slickrock help us gain elevation on steeper stretches. Above this grade we level off, passing through a fascinating landscape of low, cross-bedded Moab Tongue Sandstone, and climbing into a shallow draw. Plant life in this slickrock desert finds a toehold wherever sand and silt have collected, enduring extreme heat and drought as well as torrential downpours.

Soon our trail traverses the nearly vertical north face of a slickrock fin, clinging to the sheer cliff like a narrow catwalk. We quickly pass beneath small Frame Arch, and when we crest the fin at 1.5 miles (4840'), we are confronted with a magnificent, not-soon-to-be-forgotten sight.

Lonely Delicate Arch, 45 feet high with a 33-foot span, frames the lofty La Sal Mountains on the southeast horizon. This point is a popular destination with photographers, particularly at sunset. This beautiful arch is justifiably the most photographed feature in the park. Distant horizons also beg our attention: the extensive wall of the Book Cliffs rises above the vast desert lands on the northern horizon, and a number of lofty mesas foreground the La Sal Mountains in the southeast. The maze of spires and fins of the Fiery Furnace lie closer at hand in the west, across a white slickrock tableland composed of the Moab Tongue Sandstone. Take notice of that rock's jointed nature, a result of stresses imposed by the upward-bulging Salt Valley Anticline. Thick vegetation grows where soil has collected in each of the north-south-trending joints.

A small bowl lies below Delicate Arch, and below it unseen cliffs plummet into the depths of Winter Camp Wash. Farther south lies Cache Valley.

Its floor rises gently southward, past stark hills of Mancos Shale, which grades into the red shales of the Chinle Formation. Above, ledgy cliffs of Wingate Sandstone rise steeply to a broad tableland composed of the Kayenta Formation, sparsely clad in shrubs and pygmy forest. The latter three rock units will be familiar to visitors of Capitol Reef National Park, but they are prominent in Arches only in the lower Salt Wash area.

Towering Elephant Butte, the high point of the park, rears above the Kayenta tableland. We see the opening of South Window in the distance. Colorful greenish slopes of the Cedar Mountain Formation and Brushy Basin Shale dominate our view into Salt Valley to the southwest. We may also notice that an alcove is forming in the fin to our west, directly opposite the small alcove we passed before reaching Frame Arch.

From Delicate Arch, return the way you came. ■

Hike 31. Delicate Arch Viewpoint

Distance	1.4 miles round trip
Elevation gain	250′
Average hiking time	30 to 45 minutes
Difficulty rating	2
Child rating	2
Best seasons	April through mid-June; mid-September through November
Hazards	Slickrock scrambling; steep dropoffs

Driving to the trailhead

Follow driving directions for Hike 26 to reach Arches National Park, then follow the paved park road generally north for 11.2 miles to the junction with the spur road to Wolfe Ranch, Delicate Arch Trailhead, and Delicate Arch Viewpoint.

Turn right here onto the paved road and drive 1.2 miles to the short spur road leading to the parking area at Wolfe Ranch, then continue straight ahead (east) for another 1 mile to the road's end at the spacious Delicate Arch Viewpoint parking area.

Introduction

Park visitors without the time or energy to hike to Delicate Arch can nevertheless enjoy a fine view of that beautiful span from an unusual perspective by following the short trail from the Delicate Arch Viewpoint parking area in Cache Valley. The trail crosses much slickrock, and a sheer cliff plunges 200 feet down from the trail's end, so caution is advised and parents must closely supervise children.

Description

From the roadend (4350′), the gravel trail heads east for about 100 yards to an interpretive display and a view of Delicate Arch. A longer, also graveled trail follows immediately east of the course of a reclaimed road (which formerly led to a ridgetop viewpoint) to a broad saddle at 0.3 mile (4450′). Here we mount slickrock and begin steadily ascending. The trail ahead winds amid scattered junipers and Mormon Tea. A variety of shrubs and spring wildflowers is near as we climb a boulder-littered hill atop the Salt Wash Sandstone member of the Morrison Formation. We ascend through the red rocks of the Tidwell member, then the slickrock slopes of the Moab Tongue, following cairns as we do.

Our route ends at 0.7 mile (4600') at the brink of sheer cliffs that plunge 200 feet into Winter Camp Wash, its cottonwood-lined course disappearing into the slickrock to the northeast. Rock Setee, a prominent sandstone monolith, juts above the wash. Above the north walls of the canyon lies a slickrock bowl stretching to the skyline. Isolated stone pinnacles and solitary Delicate Arch, 0.4 mile away, decorate the bowl. The graceful, aptly named Delicate Arch is the symbol of the park, and it adorns roadside signs, Utah state license plates, and covers of numerous park publications.

After enjoying this unusual perspective of Delicate Arch, we backtrack to the trailhead.   ■

Hike 32. Sand Dune and Broken Arches

Distance	1.6 miles round trip to Broken Arch; 1.8 miles round trip to Sand Dune and Broken arches
Elevation gain	140'
Average hiking time	30 to 40 minutes
Difficulty rating	2
Child rating	1 to 2
Best seasons	April through mid-June; mid-September through November
Hazards	Negligible

Driving to the trailhead

Follow driving directions for Hike 26 to reach Arches National Park, then follow the paved park road generally north and northwest for 15.7 miles to the signed trailhead on the right (east) side of the road.

Introduction

This pleasant jaunt offers access to two lovely arches, and boasts far-flung vistas and a curious distribution of desert plants. Each plant in this high desert country has certain environmental requirements, and their distribution depends on local environmental conditions. On this short hike, we'll notice that grasses and certain shrubs thrive in deep, well-drained soils; on slickrock, where the soil cover is shallow, shrubs such as blackbrush dominate; and at the very foot of the fins of Devils Garden and Fiery Furnace, where bedrock lies just below the surface, pinyon and juniper grow.

Description

From the trailhead (5180'), our sandy trail strikes out northeast, below an impressive array of salmon-hued slickrock fins. Blackbrush, Indian ricegrass and Mormon Tea dominate the vegetation in the broad flat between Devils Garden to our north and the fins of Fiery Furnace above us in the south. After skirting the south edge of the flat for 100 yards, we reach the trail to Sand Dune Arch on our right and the longer trail to Broken Arch on our left.

Turning right, we plunge into the fins via a narrow crack. We work our way southeast up the small, sand-floored joint flanked by tall, steep-walled fins. Just 200 yards from the junction, we reach the small dune beneath the arch that gave this span its name. This small opening, 30 feet long and only 8 feet high, is formed entirely within the Entrada's Slick Rock member. This is a delightful locale, and it receives little sunshine. Narrow joints on the opposite side of the arch would be good scrambling terrain for experienced hikers.

Return to the aforementioned junction and bear right (north) onto the sandy red trail that leads 0.4 mile across the flat. Ahead, Broken Arch lies on the north margin of the flat, beyond which rises a maze of tall, colorful fins. A variety of grasses, prickly pear, blackbrush, Mormon Tea, four-wing salt-bush, and winterfat—an important winter browse for mule deer—are all found in this grassland environment. After a gentle stint across the flat, we arrive at a junction at 0.7 mile (5180'). The left fork climbs through the fins to the campground in 0.5 mile. We bear right, curving northeast along the foot of the fins.

Notice the pinyons and junipers crowding the sandy flats at the feet of the fins. Since virtually all rainwater runs off the slickrock, flats like these at the feet of the cliffs receive considerable moisture from the runoff. It is likely that slickrock also lies not far underground, capturing much of this moisture in subsurface potholes. Hence these trees have found a suitable habitat, and grow thickly and to atypical sizes. By contrast, the flat we previously tra-

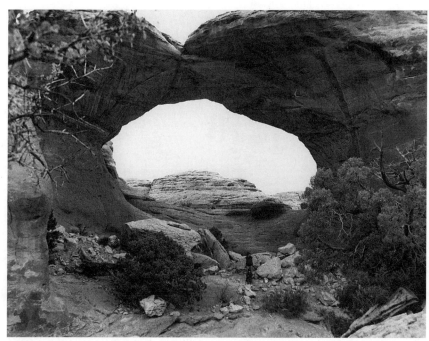

Broken Arch

versed does not support any trees; its deep soils are unable to hold adequate moisture in the root area.

Finally we dip into a slickrock gully and climb briefly to the arch at 0.8 mile (5200'). Broken Arch's opening is 43 feet high and 59 feet wide. Capped by white, wind-deposited Moab Tongue Sandstone, it is largely composed of the Slick Rock member of the Entrada Sandstone. The arch penetrates an east-west-trending fin standing well above the aforementioned gully. This arch isn't actually broken, but there is a deep notch in the caprock atop the arch. The base of the arch is littered with buff-colored boulders fallen from the Moab Tongue that caps the fin.

Through the rock-framed opening, vistas stretch from the lofty La Sals in the southeast to the Uncompahgre Plateau—site of an ancient mountain range that supplied sediments for the Arches region—on the northeast horizon. From Broken Arch we retrace our route to the trailhead. ∎

Hike 33. Devils Garden Trails

Distances	1.6 miles round trip to Landscape Arch; 4 miles round trip to Double O Arch; 5.4 miles round trip to Dark Angel; or 7.2 miles loop trip visiting all the arches and returning via the primitive trail.
Elevation gain	50' to 350'
Average hiking time	1 to 3½ hours
Difficulty rating	1 (Landscape Arch); 2 (Double O Arch and Dark Angel); 3 (for loop)
Child rating	1 (Landscape Arch); 2 (Double O Arch and Dark Angel); 3 (for loop)
Best seasons	April through mid-June; mid-September through November
Hazards	Little shade; steep dropoffs; some scrambling over slickrock required beyond Landscape Arch and on primitive loop trail

Driving to the trailhead

Follow driving directions for Hike 26 to reach Arches National Park, then follow the paved park road generally north and northwest for 17.5 miles to the spacious but often congested parking area in the loop at the end of the park road.

Introduction

Devils Garden is one of the most heavily used areas in Arches, and the reasons become apparent soon after you leave the trailhead. The area is a wonderland of standing rocks, with far-reaching and panoramic views; the first mile of the trail is wide and gravelled; and most of all, there are more readily observed arches in Devils Garden (at least nine) than in any other area of the park.

Despite the heavy use, this is one hike no one should miss. The so-called primitive trail into Fin Canyon offers hikers the chance to see more of Devils Garden, and offers a modicum of solitude for only a little extra effort. The primitive trail does require some steep slickrock scrambling, and should be attempted only by experienced hikers. The trail beyond Landscape Arch to

Double O Arch and Dark Angel is also considered a "primitive" trail and, although it crosses slickrock as well, it is easily negotiated by novice hikers.

Description

A wayside exhibit at the trailhead (5180') lists mileage to the eight arches accessed by the main trail. Our wide, gravelled trail wastes no time plunging into Devils Garden via an erosion-enlarged joint between towering, salmon-hued fins. Trees and shrubs colonize every available space where sand from the fins above has collected.

After 0.1 mile, we reach a sandy flat embraced by rock walls, where sand sagebrush, four-wing saltbush, yucca, Mormon Tea, and Indian ricegrass mass their ranks next to the trail. At 0.3 mile (5200'), the spur trail to Tunnel and Pine Tree arches forks off to the right. This smooth trail quickly descends in 50 yards to a junction, from which trails lead right (south) to Tunnel Arch, and left (north) to Pine Tree Arch. Turning right at this junction, 100 yards up a blind draw you reach a fine view of Tunnel Arch. Piercing the large, thick fin to the west high above the ground, this window-like opening is one of the better-proportioned in the park, appearing as a nearly round tunnel. The span measures 22 feet high by 27 feet wide. A smaller, even more tunnel-like arch pierces the fin above and to the left of Tunnel Arch.

• • • • • • • • • • • •
Pine Tree Arch

To reach Pine Tree Arch, head north from the junction, hugging the fins to the left while you skirt a broad flat, and then enter a blind draw. We won't get a glimpse of the arch until we reach it, but in less than 0.2 mile we're there. The angularity of the opening indicates that in the not-so-distant past, blocks have fallen from its roof and enlarged the opening. Unlike many arches in the park, the opening is at ground level. From the right perspective, the arch frames twisted pinyons and junipers in addition to the extensive Book Cliffs and nearby Crystal Arch to the northeast, and an array of domes and fins closer at hand. This span stretches 46 feet between abutments and rises 48 feet from roof to floor. Above the opening, a series of stress fractures has developed which will lead to the inevitable enlargement of the arch. Both Pine Tree and Tunnel arches lie within the Slick Rock member of the Entrada Sandstone.

• • • • • • • • • • • •

Back on the main trail, at a point 0.3 mile from the trailhead, we continue between more massive fins, soon passing a lone pinnacle—all that remains of an eroded fin. But just before reaching that spire, a look to the north reveals a tiny opening in a cliff, the beginnings of another arch. Soon

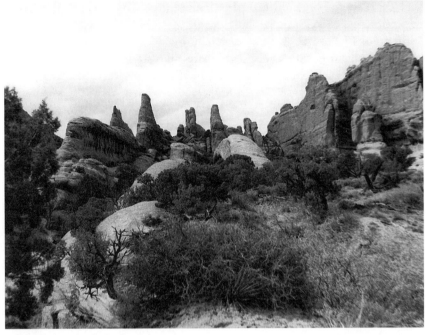

Jointed fins in Devils Garden

the trail breaks out into the open and crosses a broad flat. We might spy new arches being formed and the broken remnants of former arches in the fins to our left.

One-half mile from the previous junction, the improved segment of the trail ends, and the primitive loop trail forks at 0.8 mile (5230'). Bearing left, you quite soon reach a point just east of Landscape Arch, visible nearby in the west. This is a lovely, fragile-looking ribbon of stone, and with such an easy access trail, it is the arch that most visitors to Devils Garden come to see. Landscape Arch is an old-timer, with only a mere ribbon of stone framing its huge opening. Its fragile appearance and old age are apparent; it is possible the span will "soon" collapse. It could happen at any time, but when you compare the first known photograph of the arch, taken in 1896, its appearance has changed very little. Viewed from behind, the arch frames a fine picture of distant landscapes.

The arch was dubbed "Landscape" in 1934 by Frank Beckwith, director of the Arches National Monument Scientific Expedition. Many have claimed Landscape Arch to be the largest natural rock span in the world, but others claim that title for mighty Kolob Arch in Zion National Park. Kolob and Landscape arches were measured by two different groups from Brigham Young University in 1983 and 1984. The teams used different methods of measurement, and as one might expect, they arrived at different dimensions for each arch. The presently accepted dimensions of Landscape Arch are that the arch rises 106 feet, with a width of 306 feet, while Kolob Arch estimates range from 177 to 230 feet high and 292 to 310 feet wide. (Kolob Arch is more difficult to measure since it is inaccessible, high on a vertical wall.) It has been suggested that a standardized method of measurement be used to measure rock spans on the Colorado Plateau, but until then the controversy remains. Facts and figures aside, let us simply enjoy this exceptionally beautiful arch and marvel at its uniqueness.

Beyond Landscape Arch we must briefly follow cairns over slickrock as we climb a passageway between fins, passing very close to Wall Arch (68 feet wide by 41 feet high) after 0.1 mile. This slickrock ascent soon levels off on a juniper- and pinyon-decorated notch. In this notch, at 1.3 miles (5400'), we meet a left-forking spur trail bound for Navajo and Partition arches. Following this spur, we proceed across a shady bench and in 100 yards we reach a fork—left to Partition, right to Navajo, two markedly different spans, both well worth visiting.

• • • • • • • • • • • •

Partition Arch

The spur to Partition Arch, an interesting 0.25-mile stroll, passes through a narrow, wooded bench leading to the nearly round opening of the arch. The arch penetrates the uppermost part of a tall, desert-varnished fin, which rises about 30 feet above the arch. Viewed from the vicinity of Landscape Arch, Partition Arch seems inaccessibly high on a sheer wall, but standing in the opening we find ourselves on the edge of a cliff plummeting 100 feet or more to the east. The opening stretches 26 feet from side to side and rises 28 feet from its base. A smaller arch lies about 15 feet south, on the same wall, separated by a stone "partition." Its opening, also nearly round, is 8.5 feet wide and only 8 feet tall. The arch nicely frames views of Devils Garden and the distant Uncompahgre Plateau, across the border in Colorado.

• • • • • • • • • • •

Navajo Arch

To visit Navajo Arch, we turn left back at the junction, heading into a wooded draw between low fins. Passing an intriguing honeycombed wall, we continue under an overhang to alcove-like Navajo Arch, reached in 0.2 mile. A low fin rises immediately behind (west of) Navajo Arch and the fin it penetrates. Between the two fins is a narrow, sand-floored joint, aligned northwest to southeast, as are all fins and joints in Devils Garden. The arch is 41 feet wide at its base and 13 feet high, a nearly perfect half-circle.

• • • • • • • • • • • •

Back on the main trail at a junction 1.3 miles from the trailhead, we proceed briefly across benchland before curving to the rim above Salt Valley. We enjoy fine, expansive vistas that stretch from northwest to southeast across a vast, empty landscape. Our route then turns northwest and crosses much slickrock, at times passing atop narrow fins where faint-hearted hikers may wish to turn back. A short scramble to the west affords broad views into Salt Valley and beyond. Traversing above the abyss of magnificent Fin Canyon, we enjoy a head-on view of parallel ranks of narrow, salmon-hued fins, rising northwest and southeast above the dry wash of the wooded canyon.

At 1.7 miles, we come to another junction, just 0.4 miles from the previous one. A few yards to the right is an overlook on the rim above Fin Canyon. True to its name, large Black Arch lies in the dark, mysterious folds of the canyon.

Continuing straight from the junction, towards Double O Arch, our trail begins climbing, passing a few small arches and tunnels where scattered wallflowers enliven the stark trailside landscape with their vivid yellow blooms in spring. Still on slickrock, we make our way between fins and through groves of pinyon and juniper. Suddenly, as we cross over a jointed fin, Double O Arch comes into view; its smaller opening is partly obscured by trees.

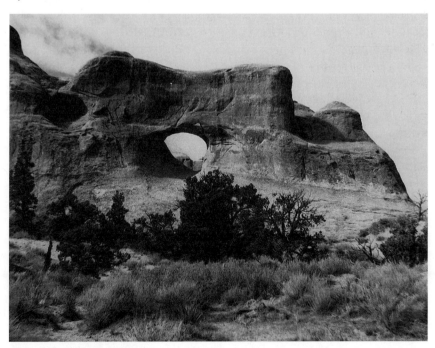

Tunnel Arch in Devils Garden

Finally, descending northwest along the top of a slickrock fin, we curve west among large pinyons and reach the foot of the larger oval opening of Double O Arch, piercing the north end of a narrow, desert-varnished fin. The top of the opening is a fine arching ribbon of stone, and a prominent tower rises north of the arch abutting the north end of the fin. The two oval arches measure 71 feet wide by 45 feet high, and 21 feet by 9 feet. Scramble around to the southwest side of the fin for the best view, framing the fins of Devils Garden.

The arch was named in 1927 by Hugh Bell, then a reporter and photographer for a Cleveland newspaper. He left an inscription on each of three arches in the park that he named, but Double O is the only name that has survived. One of his other inscriptions can be found under Tower Arch in the Klondike Bluffs. You can see the "Double O Arch" inscription in the smaller opening in the fin.

Shortly beyond the arch, the signed loop trail forks off to the right at 2.1 miles (5420'), and another trail continues west (left) for 0.6 mile to Dark Angel. Following the left fork, intermittent cairns mark our route, leading across blackbrush-dominated slopes amid pinyon and juniper. We attain a northwest-trending slickrock ridge and at once enjoy broad vistas into Salt Valley, backdropped by a broken redrock ridge and the jumbled Klondike Bluffs. Eventually we reach the foot of the tall, desert-varnished spire of Dark Angel at 2.7 miles (5450'), a solitary, remnant of an ancient fin, and the end of the trail.

From Dark Angel you have two options: either backtrack to the trailhead or, to see more of Devils Garden, backtrack just 0.6 mile to the last junction, and and turn left (northwest) onto the primitive loop trail. Following the primitive trail from that junction, we briefly drop into a woodland at the head of a draw that trends northwest. Yucca, cliffrose, alder-leaf mountain mahogany, Utah serviceberry, Mormon Tea, and Indian rice-grass keep us company as we proceed, soon curving northeast and descending the dry wash between towering fins.

Watching for cairns on this ill-defined route, we soon pass through a short narrows. When the canyon opens up, we see an arch in the fins a short distance to the north. Widely spaced cairns lead us briefly toward that arch across slickrock before curving back into the main wash. Ahead we bypass a few dry falls before heading southeast over a low rise and descending toward Fin Canyon, below in the south. Massive vertical, sometimes overhanging cliffs embrace the joints we are descending, and we must negotiate a very steep slickrock slope to proceed.

As we approach Fin Canyon, the route suddenly veers away from a narrow joint and heads north over a low slickrock fin. Proceeding over the fin, we then reach a series of narrow ledges that we must traverse above a defile to reach the floor of Fin Canyon.

About 0.2 mile downstream, an arrow sign points in both directions, indicating our route. From here we climb moderately southeast on well-defined trail. Fins in the lower canyon diminish in stature toward the east, and are now capped by the cream-colored Moab Tongue Sandstone.

As we climb generally southeast on blackbrush-clad slopes, the view back across aptly named Fin Canyon is exciting, even awe-inspiring. Ranks of parallel fins and sharp pinnacles form a sawtoothed horizon.

This climb tops out between trailside domes, and then we head south along the west edge of a brushy flat, then rise easily once again west of a group of low, eroded fins. Crystal Arch, seen through Pine Tree Arch earlier in our journey, lies among these fins east of the trail. Hiking southeast again, we may see hikers treading the improved trail in the southwest, and we soon curve southwest under an overhanging cliff as Landscape Arch appears to the west. After following the primitive trail for 2.1 miles, we turn left to retrace our route for 0.8 mile to the trailhead. ■

Hike 34. Tower Arch Trail

Distance	3.4 miles round trip
Elevation gain	450'
Average hiking time	2 to 2½ hours
Difficulty rating	3
Child rating	2 to 3
Best seasons	April through mid-June; mid-September through October
Hazards	Little shade

Driving to the trailhead

Follow driving directions for Hike 26 to reach Arches National Park, then follow the paved park road generally north and northwest for 16.2 miles to the left-branching Salt Valley Road. This road is an infrequently maintained dirt road; its surface is usually rough, although it is passable to 2WD vehicles. It should be avoided by all vehicles for a day or so following heavy rains.

After turning south from the main park road onto the descending Salt Valley Road, you begin winding down into the vast expanse of Salt Valley. Upon reaching the wash draining Salt Valley, the road describes a tight turn toward the northwest. Soon you pass between low red hills, then enter a narrow section of the wash, a dangerous place to be during heavy rains.

The road ahead soon rises over a hill, then descends onto the broad plain of the valley and follows a course northwest through the center of the 2-mile-wide valley.

After 7 usually rough miles you reach a signed junction with a 4WD road that forks left (southwest), offering drivers of 4WD vehicles and mountain bikers access to the fringes of Klondike Bluffs. Fifty yards beyond, the 2WD road to Tower Arch Trailhead also forks left. First heading west, it then curves southwest for 1 mile to the small trailhead parking area at the foot of Klondike Bluffs. This narrow dirt road is passable to drivers of most passenger vehicles.

Introduction

The jumble of white-capped redrock fins and towers known as the Klondike Bluffs, rising above the desert floor east of U.S. Highway 191, are the first exciting features visitors view enroute to Arches National Park from the north. This remote area in the far northwest corner of the park is a miniature version of Devils Garden. When "discovered" by a miner in 1922, the Klondike Bluffs were in fact dubbed Devils Garden; later, that name was applied to the area on the opposite side of Salt Valley. The bluffs take their name from the cold and windy winter conditions in the region.

This fine short hike leads to outstanding Tower Arch, and hikers should enjoy considerable solitude compared to the popular trails along the main park road. This is an ideal area in which to spend a day or more exploring hidden canyons and searching for arches.

Take this trip as a dayhike; the area is closed to overnight camping all year.

Description

The abrupt east flank of the Klondike Bluffs, with broken cliffs and towering fins, looms boldly 400 feet above the juniper-studded trailhead (5120'). Our trail will lead around the bluffs to their west side, where a maze of cracks and joints offers access into the heart of this slickrock massif. From the trailhead, we cross a red-sandy flat dotted with junipers, blackbrush and cliffrose, and then climb steeply up a band of Navajo Sandstone. This rock unit underlies the Entrada Sandstone in Arches—a narrow, discontinuous band of rock in the ridge bounding the southwest margin of Salt Valley. Its most prominent exposure in the park occurs south of The Windows Section on topographic maps as a vast region of "petrified dunes."

Topping out on a bench and proceeding south along the 5200-foot contour, we notice three prominent rock units above us: the Navajo Sandstone, and the Dewey Bridge and Slick Rock members of the Entrada Sandstone. This exposure contrasts the differing erosional characteristics of each unit, the Dewey Bridge member being the softest. This layer underlies many of the park's arches. Erosion can undercut it, leaving little or no support for the Slick Rock member above. Consequently, fractures develop and slabs spall off of fins and cliffs, leading to the development of alcoves and ultimately arches.

In spring, rockcress and Indian paintbrush enliven this otherwise drab, brushy bench. We soon leave the bench, climbing over a band of Navajo Sandstone and shortly topping out along a broad ridge at 0.5 mile (5220'), just below the contact zone where the Navajo Sandstone and the Dewey Bridge member meet. Expansive views, unobstructed by fins or trees, stretch from the extensive wall of the Book Cliffs in the northeast to the lofty 12,000-foot summits of the La Sal Mountains in the southeast. Devils Garden and its vast array of redrock fins punctuate the rim of Salt Valley east of our viewpoint, and the rolling ridges of the Abajo Mountains lie beyond legions of vast mesas in the south. This is a pleasant place to rest and soak in the vast, contrasting landscapes, seemingly untouched by the works of man.

Now we descend west on a gentle-to-moderate grade, entering a pinyon-juniper woodland. The imposing Klondike Bluffs jut skyward north of the bowl we are descending. To the south we see a jumble of balanced rocks; above them, the striking pinnacles of the Marching Men parade across the landscape.

Descending beyond the reaches of the buff-colored Navajo Sandstone, we pass into a large amphitheater-like basin, embraced on three sides by upthrusting slickrock. At 1.0 mile (4950'), the bottom of our descent, we cross two dry, sandy washes, then climb loose red sand to an arrow sign. We are now atop an exposure of the contorted Dewey Bridge member, below a solitary, desert-varnished fin composed of the Entrada's Slick Rock member. Note the contrast between these two rock units; the lower is soft and irregular, while the upper is hard and smooth. Walking to the opposite side of the small fin from the sign, we see how the comparatively soft Dewey Bridge member is eroding away from beneath the fin. Such erosion often results in slab failure above, and often contributes to the development of arches.

Presently on a northwest course, we enter the realm of the Klondike Bluffs, where upright, salmon-hued slickrock fins and spires flank our route on either side. Ahead we descend slickrock between imposing fins, and soon spy a striking double arch in an alcove on our right. We then quickly pass the opening of a former arch and pass the ill-defined trail from a 4WD road on our left. At 1.7 miles (5200'), we reach the foot of the large oval span of Tower Arch. A tall shaft of salmon-tinted slickrock rises behind the span, capped by a huge knob of white sandstone. This tower is one of the most imposing landforms in the Klondike Bluffs area, soaring above the maze of slickrock fins that dominate the scene.

Scramble up slickrock to stand amid the massive abutments of the arch and enjoy a sandstone-framed picture of the shrub-dotted parallel fins of the bluffs, with distant mesas to the southwest delineating the horizon. This arch of stone and its abutments, formed entirely within the Slick Rock member, are thicker both vertically and horizontally than many in the park.

When government surveys were conducted in the mid-1920s in the Arches region for possible designation as a national monument, the name "Devils Garden" was mistakenly placed on The Windows Section, and later it was applied to the area that still bears the name. When Arches gained National Monument status in 1929, the original Devils Garden (Klondike Bluffs) was not included within its boundaries, and it was overlooked during the surveys. Not until 1938, did Klondike Bluffs become a part of Arches, when the monument was enlarged to encompass more than 30,000 acres.

Hikers who look closely will find two inscriptions carved into Tower Arch, one each on the bases of the north and south abutments. Beneath the south abutment an inscription reads: DISCOV'D BY M. AND MRS. ALEX RING-

HOEFFER AND SONS 1922-23. Although Alexander Ringhoffer is indisputably the "discoverer" of the Klondike Bluffs area (or at least the first person to help bring the area to the public's attention), this inscription has led to controversy because the name "Ringhoffer" is misspelled and the date 1922–23 is ambiguous. Apparently Ringhoffer did not attempt to name the arch, and it is unknown who actually carved the inscription.

A much smaller inscription near the foot of the north abutment indicates the first title given to the span. It reads: MINARET BRIDGE. H.S. BELL 1927. When Frank Beckwith, leader of the Arches National Monument Scientific Expedition who named many of the park's features, imposed "Tower Arch" in 1934, he was unaware of this title. Moreover, the opening is not a bridge, since it does not span a watercourse. One lasting title bestowed by H.S. Bell is Double O Arch, which survives to this day.

From Tower Arch, retrace your steps to the trailhead. ■

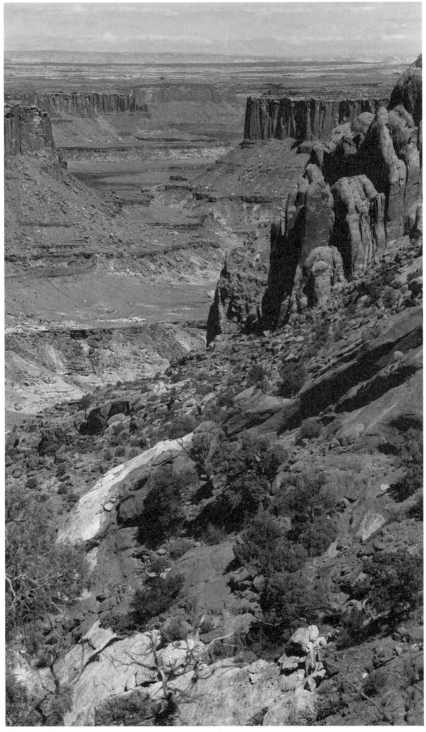

Upheaval Canyon

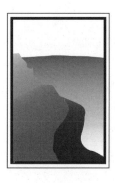

Canyonlands
National Park

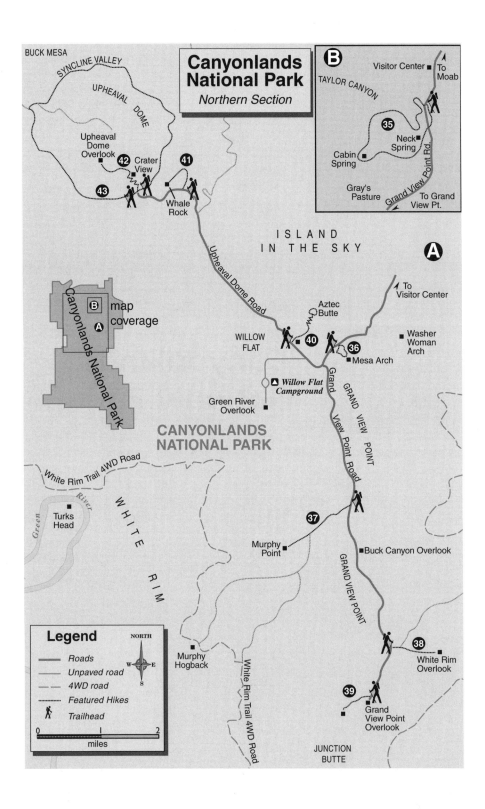

Canyonlands National Park
Northern Section

BUCK MESA

SYNCLINE VALLEY

UPHEAVAL DOME

Upheaval Dome Overlook
42 Crater View
41
43
Whale Rock

B
TAYLOR CANYON
Visitor Center ■ To Moab
35
Neck Spring
Cabin Spring
Gray's Pasture
Grand View Point Rd.
To Grand View Pt.

I S L A N D
I N   T H E   S K Y

A

Upheaval Dome Road

Canyonlands National Park

B map coverage
A

To Visitor Center

Aztec Butte
WILLOW FLAT
40
36
Mesa Arch

Washer Woman Arch

Willow Flat Campground

Green River Overlook

CANYONLANDS NATIONAL PARK

Grand View Point Road

GRAND   VIEW   POINT

White Rim Trail 4WD Road

Green River

Turks Head

W H I T E

R I M

37
Murphy Point

Buck Canyon Overlook

GRAND VIEW POINT

Legend

NORTH

— Roads
— Unpaved road
--- 4WD road
···· Featured Hikes
↟ Trailhead

W — E
S

Murphy Hogback

White Rim Trail 4WD Road

38
White Rim Overlook

39
Grand View Point Overlook

JUNCTION BUTTE

0   1   2
miles

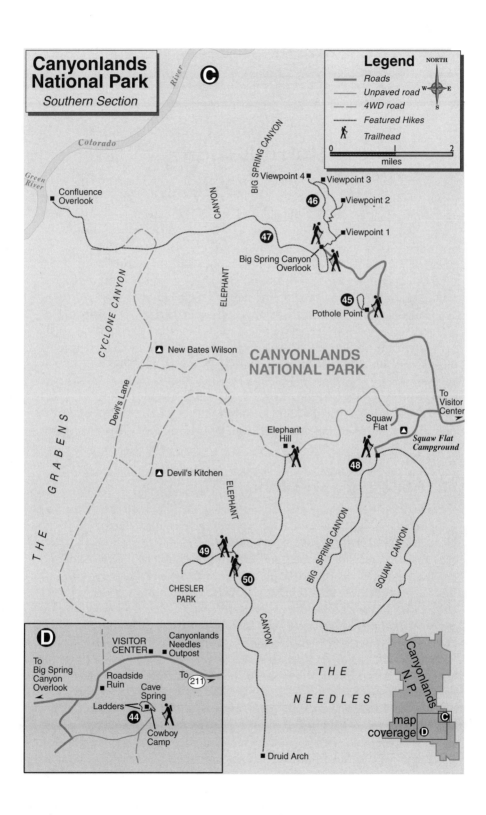

Canyonlands National Park
Southern Section

C

Legend NORTH

Roads
Unpaved road
4WD road
Featured Hikes
Trailhead

0   1   2
miles

W — E
S

River

Colorado

Green River

BIG SPRING CANYON

Confluence Overlook

CANYON

Viewpoint 4 **46** Viewpoint 3
Viewpoint 2

47 Viewpoint 1

Big Spring Canyon Overlook

ELEPHANT

CYCLONE CANYON

45
Pothole Point

New Bates Wilson

CANYONLANDS
NATIONAL PARK

Devil's Lane

To Visitor Center

THE GRABENS

Squaw Flat

Squaw Flat Campground

Elephant Hill

48

Devil's Kitchen

ELEPHANT

BIG SPRING CANYON

SQUAW CANYON

49

50

CHESLER PARK

CANYON

THE

NEEDLES

Druid Arch

D

VISITOR CENTER

Canyonlands Needles Outpost

To Big Spring Canyon Overlook

Roadside Ruin

Cave Spring

To (211)

Ladders

44

Cowboy Camp

Canyonlands N.P.

map coverage **D**

C
D

Introduction

When one tries to visualize Utah's canyon country, images of towering mesas and buttes, sheer and colorful cliffs, and yawning defiles appear in the mind's eye. Canyonlands National Park's 337,570 acres have all that and more. Two great rivers and the gaping canyons they have carved, broad and open desert flats, wooded buttes and mesas, a maze of serpentine canyons, extensive grasslands, woodlands of pinyon and juniper, a rainbow of colorful rocks, and more than 100 square miles of slickrock fins, buttes, and spires reside within the vast and remote reaches of this magnificent park.

Canyonlands is far removed from civilization, and to get to any one of its three districts you must travel many miles from primary highways. The park receives much less use than any other national park in Utah, averaging only about 500,000 visitors each year. If you wish to avoid the crowds encountered in most national parks and enjoy some of the most majestic scenery on the Colorado Plateau, Canyonlands beckons. The park consists of three separate districts—four, including the rivers. Each district is distinctly different from the others, so Canyonlands is more like three parks than one.

The Island in the Sky District

The lofty, wedge-shaped Island in the Sky mesa juts south into the vast Canyonlands basin toward the confluence of the Green and Colorado rivers. Two arms of this highland, rising more than 2000 feet above the river canyons, diverge near the southern terminus of the mesa. The western arm extends northwest to curious Upheaval Dome, then breaks away abruptly into deep and narrow canyons that yield seasonal runoff to the Green River's Labyrinth Canyon. The southern arm, aptly named Grand View Point, projecting 5 miles from its base at the Island in the Sky, ends abruptly where cliffs plunge 400 feet from its rim; an erosional outlier of the mesa, ½-square-mile Junction Butte, rises beyond. Not only is 6400-foot Junction Butte the apex of the Island District, it is one of the most prominent landmarks in all the Canyonlands basin.

The park road traverses the entire mesa system of the Island in the Sky, and turnouts located along the roadway offer far-ranging panoramas of hundreds of square miles of rugged canyons, plunging cliffs, vast desert basins, mesas and their isolated buttes, and lofty mountain ranges. Vistas are what the Island is noted for, and visitors will not be disappointed as they gaze over the entire length and breadth of Canyonlands National Park and beyond.

The Needles District

Many visitors consider The Needles to be the most beautiful district in the park. The vast reaches of this large district contain a maze of serpentine canyons and tens of square miles of banded slickrock spires, fins, cliffs, buttes, bluffs, and knolls, all colored in shades of white and red, and composed of one of the older rock formations in Canyonlands—the Cedar Mesa Sandstone. Vertical relief in this jumble of standing rocks varies from a few feet to as much as 800 feet.

A number of canyons cut far into the heart of The Needles, and many of them are corridors through which foot trails and 4WD trails pass. But only one canyon has carved a drainage completely through The Needles District and beyond park boundaries—Salt Creek. Salt Creek is the principal drainage in the district, gathering its seasonal waters high on Salt Creek Mesa and winding north and northwest for more than 20 miles to the Colorado River.

North of The Needles proper is a landscape of an entirely different character. Slickrock still abounds, but the relief is minor, save for a few abyssal defiles. The shape of the land is relatively uniform, with only low knolls and knobs of Cedar Mesa Sandstone jutting above it. But there are also broad reaches where there is no slickrock, occupied by brushy flats, scattered pinyon and juniper woodlands, and wide, grassy pockets that lend a bucolic tone to the landscape.

Stretching west from The Needles to the brink of the Colorado River canyon is a unique landscape called The Grabens, a series of closely spaced, narrow, parallel valleys trending northeast-southwest. The valleys are clad in grasses and scattered desert shrubs, and are embraced by broken cliffs, composed primarily of Cedar Mesa Sandstone, which rise as much as 400 feet from the valley floors. These unusual graben valleys are the result of the subsidence of blocks of the earth's crust along a series of faults.

From the rim of the Colorado River, broken cliffs and ruined walls plummet 1000 feet or more into the narrow gorge the river has carved. The oldest rocks in Canyonlands are exposed here in the depths of this great canyon.

The Maze District

Many people have gazed at the labyrinth of colorful slickrock canyons and the tall pillars of red rock in the Maze District from overlooks in the Island and Needles districts, but very few have braved the treacherous 4WD roads and long hiking trails to reach that remote and beautiful landscape. To learn more about the Maze District, which is beyond the scope of this book, obtain a copy of the comprehensive guidebook *Utah's National Parks*, by the author, published by Wilderness Press.

Plants and animals of Canyonlands

Canyonlands is a vast arid region ranging in elevation from 3720 feet in Cataract Canyon to 6987 feet atop Cedar Mesa in the Needles District. Mean annual precipitation of 8.05 inches at the Island in the Sky and 8.63 inches at The Needles attest to the region's aridity. At first glance the landscape appears to be a barren expanse of rock and sand, but plants grow in nearly every place where even the slightest amount of soil has collected. They are, however, typically sparse due to competition for the meager moisture and nutrients available. In Canyonlands 429 species of plants have been identified.

In southeast Utah the pinyon-juniper woodland typically occupies only the highest mesas, where the soil is shallow and rainfall is greater than in the canyons and open desert. But in Canyonlands, seemingly regardless of elevation, pinyon and juniper take root wherever there is much slickrock. They obtain their moisture by growing near, and sometimes in, slickrock, extending their roots into cracks and joints in the bedrock where moisture collects.

Desert-scrub communities dominate park vegetation and the distribution of their species is determined not only by soil depth but by soil competition and mineral content. Blackbrush, a hardy, slow-growing shrub and an important food source for bighorn sheep, is a member of this community. It is ubiquitous in the park, growing at most elevations except in the inner gorges of the rivers. Blackbrush prefers mostly clay soils that do not generally exceed 2 feet in depth; moisture trapped in the bedrock beneath this shallow soil cover nurtures this shrub. Sandy sites in the scrublands host sand sagebrush, wavyleaf oak, and three species of yucca: Harriman, narrowleaf, and the large Datil yucca.

Only a scattering of coarse shrubs inhabit the lower elevations of the park, discouraged by poor soil cover and very little moisture. These shrubs are a dull gray and blend with their surroundings when viewed from a distance, lending a barren appearance to the landscape. Shadscale and Torrey ephedra are the dominant species.

Some of the largest shrubs in the park grow near grasslands and on benches in washes, particularly in the Needles District, occasionally forming impenetrable thickets. One of the most common of these shrubs is big sagebrush, distinguished by its gray, fragrant foliage. Rabbitbrush is also a quite common colonizer of disturbed sites along washes and roadsides. Several species of this shrub grow in Canyonlands, typically characterized by green stems, long, narrow, green leaves, and clusters of yellow flowers that bloom in autumn. Greasewood, a thorny shrub with fleshy leaves, and four-wing saltbush grow on the most alkaline sites. The latter takes its descriptive name from the shape of its fruit and the salty taste of its foliage.

Grasslands occupy the areas of deepest soil cover in the park. Most shrubs are unable to gather enough moisture to survive in deep soils, despite their deep root systems. Grasses typically have shallow, spreading root systems that take advantage of even the lightest rainfall.

The Needles District and the Island in the Sky mesa are both dominated by grasslands. Although the pinyon-juniper vegetation community commonly prevails in high elevation areas, soft and velvety grasses spread over the deep soils of the 6000-foot Island mesa. However, nearly 100 years of grazing in the grasslands of Canyonlands have had a serious impact upon native grasses. Wherever overgrazing or other disturbance has occurred, exotic plants, such as cheatgrass and Russian thistle (tumbleweed), have altered the makeup of the park's grassy spreads, particularly in the Needles District—Chesler Park, upper Salt Creek, and The Grabens.

The canyons host their own unique assemblage of plants. Where subsurface moisture is available in the canyons and along the rivers, a narrow ribbon of green riparian foliage grows vigorously. Fremont cottonwood is the dominant tree, most often quite large, with a spreading crown and roundish leaves that flutter in the slightest breeze.

Lanceleaf cottonwood, a hybrid between the narrowleaf cottonwood of the Rocky Mountains and the Fremont cottonwood of the Southwest, also grows in riparian areas, primarily in the Needles District. These trees offer shade to desert-weary travelers, and they are a sure sign of moisture. They take up gallons of water from the evening through the morning hours, and if one is unfortunate enough to be dying of thirst, one can dig into the sand of a dry wash near a cottonwood tree and likely find water. Only one other native riparian tree occurs in Canyonlands, the willow, of which there are three species. The exotic tamarisk, introduced to the Southwest more than 100 years ago from Eurasia as an ornamental and for erosion control, has been so successful in its new habitat that it is rapidly spreading up each tributary of the Green and Colorado rivers and vigorously supplanting the native cottonwoods and willows.

Douglas-fir and ponderosa pine are perhaps the most unusual trees found in these arid, high-desert canyons. They form isolated stands, rather than forests, in the most sheltered sites in the upper elevations of the canyons.

Even in a land so dominated by naked stone, heat and drought, the canyons nevertheless host verdant oases called hanging gardens. Hanging gardens occur wherever constant moisture issues from a canyon wall or a cliff, most often where a permeable sandstone layer overlies an impermeable stratum. Where only marginal moisture is available in a hanging garden, mosses and occasional maidenhair fern thrive, but where moisture is plentiful, water-lovers such as scarlet monkey flower and miniature columbine join these plants.

The fragrance and delicate color of wildflowers are integral parts of the Canyonlands experience. Here in the high desert, wildflowers are typically widely scattered; they include not only flowering herbs but showy shrubs as well. In some of the higher reaches of the canyons and in the pinyon-juniper woodland you may find the climbing vine clematis, or virgin's bower, easily recognized by its creamy white flowers in spring and fluffy white seed heads in autumn. Other particularly common wildflowers include milkvetches, jimson weed, groundsels, tansy-aster, evening primrose, goldenrod, Wyoming paintbrush, longleaf phlox, yellow sweetclover, penstemon, pepper-grass, and broom snakeweed, a low, clump-forming shrub that is very common throughout most of the park. It is identified by its narrow leaves and a profusion of tiny yellow blossoms that bloom in late summer, but the dried flowers often persist through much of the year.

Various cacti, including claret-cup, prickly-pear, and fishhook cactus, are also found throughout most elevations of the park. Their delicate blooms are among the largest and most showy in the park. There are dozens of other beautiful wildflowers throughout Canyonlands, and the visitor will find lists of currently blooming plants at both the Island and Needles visitor centers to aid identification.

Just as plants are restricted in their range by environmental requirements, so are many of the animals in Canyonlands. Some animals range throughout the park, and some visit the area only seasonally, particularly birds. Some animals in the park are predators, feeding either on other animals or on insects, while others depend on plants for both food and shelter.

Desert animals have adapted to the rigors of life in this arid region by their efficient use of resources, and their mobility permits them to escape the searing desert heat. For example, Ord's kangaroo rat is primarily nocturnal and it rarely drinks water. Instead, this desert rodent obtains moisture through metabolism of its primary food source—seeds. Lizards and snakes, being cold-blooded, warm themselves on rocks during the day, but retreat into the shade of a boulder or burrow when they become too warm. Blacktail jackrabbits and desert cottontails have developed an interesting means of coping with desert heat: their long ears are laced with myriad blood vessels, which help them to dissipate body heat, as well as helping them to detect predators.

Many birds are restricted to specialized habitats in Canyonlands. Cliffs and canyons host their own distinct avifauna. Hikers in the canyons often hear the melancholy, descending call of the canyon wren, but these tiny birds are not readily observed. The rock wren perches on rocky ledges and also has a distinctive song. The white-throated swift and the violet-green swallow, soaring at high speeds among the cliffs, evoke envy in all who have ever desired to fly. Cliff swallows build their mud- and-plant nests in rows, usually beneath an overhang or in an alcove, not unlike Ancestral Puebloan cliff dwellings and granaries.

Other birds, such as the turkey vulture, raven, and golden eagle, range throughout the park, soaring on thermal updrafts in search of prey or carrion. Birds such as the scrub and pinyon jays, horned lark, mountain bluebird, blue-gray gnatcatcher, kestrel, Audubon's warbler, mourning dove, and western meadow lark are common on the mesas, in grasslands, and in pinyon-juniper woodlands.

Lizards are also frequently observed denizens of the desert. Gray and red leopard lizards and green collared lizards are common in the lower elevations of the park. These reptiles feed on their smaller relatives as well as insects. Collared lizards are fascinating to watch when they run swiftly on their hind legs. Other common lizards include the fast-running whiptail, the small side-blotched and tree lizards, and the western fence swift.

Snakes are not particularly common in Canyonlands, but there are two species some hikers might encounter. The gopher snake is the larger, attaining a length of up to 5 feet. These large snakes are harmless, and help to control the rodent population. The midget faded rattlesnake is one snake hikers may wish they don't encounter. This straw-colored snake rarely exceeds 2 feet in length. It is not aggressive and is uncommon, but its rattle is small enough that it may not be heard by hikers. This rattler is usually found near grasslands and shrublands, but it can range throughout the park.

Most rodents and mammals in the park are either nocturnal or active only in the early morning and evening hours. At least seven species of bats inhabit the park, frequently seen around dusk as they emerge in search of insects. Although beavers, porcupines, and badgers are rarely seen, evidence of their handiwork abounds. Throughout the park hikers will find the large burrows of the badger and trees stripped of their bark by the porcupine.

Bobcats and coyotes range throughout the park, and it is possible that mountain lions visit the area in search of their primary food source, mule deer, which are widespread in Canyonlands, ranging from the rivers to the mesas. Perhaps the most exciting large mammal to observe in the park is the desert bighorn sheep. They range throughout Canyonlands, but the largest and most stable herd lives in the Island District, where there are an estimated 130-180 animals. Though infrequently seen, bighorns may be observed below the rim of the Island in the Sky mesa, where they display amazing agility on seemingly sheer cliffs. In the Needles District they reside in the lower reaches of the canyons and along the inner gorge of the Colorado River.

Encroachment upon bighorn range by humans is their greatest threat to survival. It is imperative that park visitors not approach bighorn sheep, but instead observe them from a distance. Bighorn-sheep observation forms are available at the park visitor centers; if you observe a sheep, the sighting should be reported to the park staff, to help researchers gain more knowledge of the bighorn's activities.

When you visit Canyonlands, take the time to observe the plants and animals, and some of their unique relationships with one another and with their environment. A national park is an excellent setting in which to observe nature largely free of human manipulation, and we must do our best not to disrupt the delicate balance among plants, animals, and a healthy, undisturbed environment.

Interpretive activities and campgrounds in Canyonlands

Each district in Canyonlands except the Maze has a visitor center offering interpretive displays and programs, books and maps for sale, and interpretive pamphlets. In Moab you can also purchase books and maps at the Moab Interagency Information Center, located at Center and Main streets. An entrance fee is collected at visitor centers in the Needles and Island districts, allowing entrance into the park for seven consecutive days.

At the Island in the Sky visitor center, rangers on duty can answer your questions about the district, issue backcountry use permits for backpackers and four-wheel drivers and mountain bikers using any of the 20 campsites in 10 locations on the White Rim Trail 4WD road, and help visitors make the most of their stay in the park. This visitor center also sells books and maps, and offers interpretive exhibits and free brochures on self-guided trails, campgrounds, and various aspects of park natural history. Business hours are 8 A.M.–4:30 P.M., with extended hours in the summer.

Self-guided trails in the Island District include the Neck Spring Trail (Hike 35), the Mesa Arch Trail (Hike 36), and the Crater View Trail (Hike 42). Evening campfire programs are held from spring through fall at the campfire circle at Willow Flat Campground. Schedules of interpretive activities in the district are posted at the visitor center.

The Willow Flat Campground is the only camping area available to visitors on the Island mesa. This pleasant campground (6050') features 12 sites set on a bench above the mesa rim, shaded by a thick woodland of pinyon and juniper. Views are excellent from the campground, including distant panoramas of the Canyonlands basin and close-up views of the sheer Wingate Sandstone cliffs that bound the mesa and the Navajo Sandstone domes that crown its rim. Wildflowers decorate the campground from spring through fall, including cryptantha, yucca, and broom snakeweed. Campers must bring their own water, and there is no fee here. Visitors are advised to arrive early, especially during the Easter, Memorial Day, and Labor Day holidays, as the campsites are on a first-come basis.

Only 14.6 miles from the Island visitor center is Dead Horse Point State Park, which offers a fine view of the Colorado River gorge, a 21-site campground with water, a visitor center and a picnic area. A fee is charged to enter the park and to use the campground.

There are two established picnic sites on the Island. One is at the end of the road at the Upheaval Dome Trailhead, in a pinyon-juniper woodland beneath the contorted rocks of the dome. The other lies 1 mile short of the Grandview Point roadend at the Gooseberry and White Rim Overlook Trailhead. This site rests on the slickrock edge of the mesa. Only a scattering of pinyons and junipers shade the site, but vistas are far-ranging and panoramic.

The Needles visitor center offers books, maps, information on weather and trail conditions, and backcountry use permits. Business hours are 8 A.M.–4:30 P.M., with extended hours in the summer.

Campfire programs in the Needles District are conducted several nights a week at the campfire circle in Squaw Flat Campground A. Self-guided trails in the district include Cave Spring (Hike 44), Pothole Point (Hike 45), and the Slickrock Trail (Hike 46). Guided hikes also follow these trails, plus parts of the Squaw Flat trail system. Schedules of activities are posted at the visitor center and at the bulletin board at Squaw Flat Trailhead A.

There is one campground in the Needles District, separated into Squaw Flat Campground A and Squaw Flat Campground B, along the west edge of Squaw Flat. They serve as trailheads for most of the trails in the district. Squaw Flat Campground A features 16 sites nestled against a long slickrock ridge, shaded by pinyon and juniper. Views from the campground are magnificent, stretching over the grassy expanse of Squaw Flat to the comb-like ridges of The Needles and a host of colorful slickrock buttes, including Woodenshoe Arch, North Six-shooter Peak, lofty Cathedral Butte and forested Horse Mountain.

Campground B, with 10 campsites, is similar in setting to Campground A in that most sites are set back against the slickrock and are shaded by pinyon and juniper. These sites lack Campground A's panoramic views but provide campers more intimate association with the immediate surroundings of low domes and slickrock knolls. Water is available at either campground, and a fee is charged. Each site includes a picnic table and fire grill, and there are toilets in each campground.

The Canyonlands Needles Outpost, located on a spur road near the park boundary, offers ample facilities and services for park visitors and is open all year. This privately owned facility offers a general store, gasoline, propane, baked goods, grill (open 11 A.M.–2 P.M.), showers, camping supplies, maps and books. A fee campground features 23 sites with water.

Reservations for campsites and two group-camping areas are accepted. Arrangements can be made there for guided 4WD tours and scenic flights out of Moab.

There are two picnic areas in the Needles District. One lies alongside the Scenic Drive near the Pothole Point Trail, on a slickrock highland offering expansive vistas. The other is at the Elephant Hill Trailhead at the head of a box canyon, shaded by a woodland of pinyon and juniper.

For those who prefer guided 4WD tours in Canyonlands or float trips on the Green and Colorado rivers, there are 13 guide services from which to choose in Moab. Moab also offers a variety of services to meet the needs of all park visitors. Moab, Monticello, and Green River, Utah, all offer groceries, gas, and lodging, plus several private campgrounds. Other campgrounds are available on nearby national-forest land, and visitors are also free to camp in existing campsites on national-forest and Bureau of Land Management lands. Everyone should attempt to minimize their impact on our priceless and irreplaceable public lands.

For more information:

Moab Headquarters Office
Canyonlands National Park
2282 South West Resource Blvd.
Moab, UT 84532
(435) 719-2313
(435) 259-7164 (for recorded information)

Monticello Office
32 South 1st East
Monticello, UT 84534
(435) 587-2737

Island District
(435) 259-4712

Needles District
(435) 259-4711

Visit the Canyonlands website at http://www.nps.gov/cany.

For information about Canyonlands Needles Outpost, contact:

Tracey Napoleone and Gary Knecht
P.O. Box 1107
Monticello, UT 84535
(435) 979-4007

Hiking in Canyonlands

The Island District

Most visitors to the Island District use the park only for a day, driving the park road to scenic overlooks and perhaps hiking some of the mesa-top trails. Except for these short, day-use trails atop the mesa, most trails in the 150,000-acre Island in the Sky District are very rugged and demanding, and virtually all the district's backcountry trails plunge steeply over the great cliff band that nearly encircles the mesa. Although these trails are downhill all the way, they are rough and rocky, and descend 1000 feet or more to the White Rim bench far below. The trails are shadeless and mostly waterless, and are quite rigorous on the return trip to the mesa. The Syncline Loop Trail (Hike 43) is the only trail in this book that descends below the rim, and is a unique backcountry trail in that surface water is available in some years, and it is partially shaded by pinyons, junipers, and cottonwoods.

Novice hikers and others who simply don't have the time, energy, or inclination to follow the longer trails below the rim have eight short but highly rewarding mesa-top trails from which to choose (Hikes 35-42). These trails sample all aspects of the mesa landscape, from arches to buttes, from grasslands to pinyon-juniper woodlands, Ancestral Puebloan granaries, and the sweeping panoramas for which the Island is famous.

Especially during spring, tiny, biting gnats will annoy you wherever you travel in the Island District, and mosquitoes can be a nuisance along rivers.

The Needles District

The Needles District contains the greatest concentration of trails in Canyonlands. This is a hiking district, and most of its visitors (who annually average over 150,000) are hikers. As in most Utah national parks, novice and casual hikers will find short and easy trails near the primary park road. The longer trails aren't particularly strenuous, but do entail much up and down hiking. Some longer trails in the district involve following cairns over slickrock and climbing ladders on steep cliffs.

The most popular trails in Canyonlands, as well as the greatest concentration of trails, are in the vicinity of Squaw Flat Campground A. From this trail network you can construct a variety of rewarding and highly scenic loop trips in the heart of The Needles.

The optimum seasons for hiking in Canyonlands National Park are much the same as in other Utah national parks. See "Hiking Seasons" in the "Hiking Utah's desert parks" section of the introduction.

While most hikers try to limit their impact while traveling through the park's backcountry, many will be lured off the main trails to gain a better view of an arch, a rock-writing panel, some Ancestral Puebloan ruins, or a particularly beautiful wildflower or animal. When traveling off-trail, try to walk over slickrock or in drainage courses as much as possible to avoid damaging the cryptobiotic crust and other coarse but fragile.

Summary of park regulations pertinent to dayhiking

Following is an abbreviated list of park regulations pertinent to dayhiking in Canyonlands National Park. See the section "Hiking Utah's desert parks" for information that will help you to reduce your impact on the fragile desert ecosystem. (For more information on backpacking in Canyonlands, obtain a copy of the comprehensive guidebook *Utah's National Parks,* by the author, published by Wilderness Press.)

- **Pets.** Pets are not allowed in the backcountry, including inside 4WD vehicles. Pets are allowed only on paved or 2WD roads and in frontcountry campgrounds. They must be on a leash at all times when outside your vehicle.

- **Backcountry sanitation.** Backpackers and dayhikers are required to bury waste in a cathole 6 to 8 inches deep, at least 300 feet from water, dry washes, alcoves, rock shelters, campsites, and archaeological sites. All used toilet paper, sanitary products, disposable diapers, etc., must be packed out. (Self-sealing plastic bags should be used.)

- **Water use regulations.**

  Swimming, bathing, and immersing human bodies in water sources are prohibited, except in the Green and Colorado rivers, and the section of Salt Creek that is open to vehicle use.

  Rinsing dishes or other equipment directly in water sources is prohibited, except in the Green and Colorado rivers.

  A water source may not be emptied or depleted for human use. ■

Hikes 35-43: Island in the Sky District

Hike 35. Neck Spring Loop Trail

Distance	5.3 miles loop trip
Elevation gain	450 feet
Average hiking time	2½ to 3 hours
Difficulty rating	3
Child rating	3
Best seasons	April through mid-June; mid-September through October
Hazards	Steep dropoffs; little shade

Driving to the trailhead

The trails of the Island District are easily reached via the paved park road, which branches off from Utah 313 near Dead Horse Point State Park.

Prominently signed Utah 313 branches southwest from U.S. 191 about 20.5 miles south of Crescent Junction and Interstate 70, and 9 miles northwest of Moab. Signs list mileage to Dead Horse Point State Park and Canyonlands National Park, and warn that no services are available ahead. Park visitors should be sure to have a full tank of gas and an ample water supply.

Follow this steadily ascending, paved, two-lane road generally southwest, then south for 14.2 miles to a junction with the left-branching road to Dead Horse Point State Park. Continue straight ahead at that junction and enter Canyonlands National Park after another 4.4 miles, 18.6 miles from U.S. 191. At 19.7 miles you reach the park entrance station, and at 20.8 miles is the Island visitor center.

The mesa becomes increasingly narrow as you descend past the visitor center, soon reaching a prominently signed spur road after another 0.5 mile, forking left and ending in 0.1 mile at the parking area at Shafer Canyon Overlook, the starting point for both the Neck Spring Loop Trail and the short Shafer Canyon Viewpoint Trail.

Introduction

This fine dayhike surveys much of the varied scenery and environments on and near the Island in the Sky mesa. Not only will hikers enjoy an intimate association with the Island mesa landscape, but far-reaching views help to put the Island into perspective in the larger scheme of Canyonlands. The hike also allows a glimpse into the bygone days of cattle and sheep ranching on the mesa, when the trickling waters of Neck and Cabin springs offered some of the few watering sources for grazing stock.

Description

Our day trip begins at the south end of the parking (5820'), branching right (west) from the Shafer Canyon Viewpoint Trail. We start a counterclockwise loop by first dropping quickly west away from the rim to the park road, crossing it via a crosswalk, and resuming our trail walk west, following cairns across a pinyon- and juniper-studded bench. Soon, an old road descends from the north to join our trail at 0.2 mile (5700'). At one time, this road offered ranchers access to the springs that lie ahead. Our trail then descends steadily for a short time, after which we reach the floor of a shallow basin at the head of Taylor Canyon, the primary drainage of the Island in the Sky mesa. The trail ahead winds south through the basin, first passing below the narrow isthmus of The Neck and then beneath a colorful Navajo Sandstone cliff.

Colorful seasonal wildflowers adorn the floor of the basin. Hikers must be sure to stay on the trail so as not to damage the well-developed cryptobiotic crust. In a pinyon-juniper woodland we curve into a shady alcove with a mossy seepline. A few minor ups and downs ensue, and we soon contour into another, deeper alcove, where seeps nurture abundant water-loving vegetation. A sheer cliff of Navajo Sandstone, streaked with red iron minerals and darkened by desert varnish, soars 200 feet behind the alcove. Cars on the road above can be heard but not seen, and we will soon be out of earshot of tourist traffic.

The trail ahead curves into more alcoves, and finally we reach the largest alcove thus far, crossing the often-damp wash below it at 1.5 miles (5660') that drains Neck Spring. Wildrose, Gambel oak, and even small Fremont cottonwoods crowd the banks of the wash. Immediately beyond the crossing a short trail forks left, climbing amid Gambel oak and juniper to an old watering trough, a remnant of the days of cattle- and sheep-grazing on the mesa.

Our trail descends north, closely following the wash downstream before contouring northwest above it, continuing our circuit around the scalloped headwaters of Taylor Canyon. The trail ahead undulates over sandy slopes amid scattered pinyon and juniper, blackbrush, and clumps of ground-hugging wavyleaf oak. In season, tall lupine, haplopappus, and scarlet gilia enliven the sandy hillside, from which we obtain fine views over cliff-bound upper Taylor Canyon and behind us to the narrow gap of The Neck.

About midway between Neck and Cabin springs, a 40-yard spur trail leaves the main route on our right, leading to a superb view into the rugged maw of Taylor Canyon. There is an abundance of cryptobiotic crust here, so stick to the trail. The main trail ahead follows a ledge of the Kayenta Formation as it bends into two more alcoves. Soon, as we approach the deep amphitheater from which Cabin Spring issues, we pass a dilapidated fence, then the remains of an old log cabin, likely a cowboy line shack.

As we hop across the damp wash draining Cabin Spring at 3.0 miles (5600'), we may notice an abrupt change in the trailside flora. Fremont barberry, wild rose, rabbitbrush, Gambel oak, and a thick turf of grasses all thrive along the moist banks of the wash. It is likely we will see the tracks of bighorn sheep, mule deer, and coyote here, as they take advantage of this perennial spring, one of few near the mesa top.

The trail ahead climbs moderately, quite soon passing an old log corral, then climbs up a draw to the west before mounting a slickrock slope of Navajo Sandstone. Cairns guide us to the rim of the mesa, where we curve south and stroll along the rim high above the oak-clad draw below Cabin Spring. We shortly reach a long water trough at 3.5 miles (5880'), where the trail begins to curve eastward. Water pumped up from Cabin Spring filled the trough for ranchers' stock prior to the park's establishment.

A pleasant mesa-top stroll east ensues, through stands of pinyon and juniper, the grasslands of Grays Pasture, and long stretches of slickrock, where the route is indicated by widely spaced cairns.

Eventually we cross the park road at 4.5 miles (5760'), then go north on an old roadbed, east of the park road in a pinyon-juniper woodland. This easy downhill stint allows us to enjoy far-flung vistas, stretching west beyond gaping Taylor Canyon to the distant San Rafael Swell on the far horizon, seen beyond 50 miles of mesas and desert incised by innumerable invisible canyons. When our trail reaches the Shafer Trail Overlook at 5.0 miles (5820'), we enjoy broad views of the Shafer Trail 4WD road switchbacking down the cliff into South Fork Shafer Canyon.

Descending easily to The Neck, we pass an old log drift fence once used to contain cattle and sheep on the Island in the Sky mesa, then climb gently amid scattered pinyon and juniper to complete the circuit at the trailhead at 5.3 miles. ■

Hike 36. Mesa Arch Loop Trail

Distance	0.5 mile loop trail
Elevation gain	80'
Average hiking time	20 to 30 minutes
Difficulty rating	1
Child rating	1
Best seasons	April through mid-June; mid-September through October
Hazards	Steep cliffs behind Mesa Arch

Driving to the trailhead

Follow driving directions for Hike 35 to reach the Island visitor center, then continue south on the park road for another 6.1 miles to the signed Mesa Arch parking area on the left (east) side of the road.

Introduction

This easy and popular self-guided nature trail passes a typical array of mesa-top vegetation and leads to Mesa Arch, a small but beautiful span formed in the Navajo Sandstone at the very rim of the mesa. The arch is a photographer's delight, as it frames a dramatic picture of the rugged Colorado River canyon and the lofty summits of the La Sal Mountains.

A pamphlet available at the trailhead describes the diverse plant life along the trail, and gives hikers a better understanding of hardy desert flora.

Description

Our short, popular jaunt begins at the edge of the Grays Pasture grasslands (6120'), where we have a fine view of Aztec Butte to the west and the peaks of the Henry Mountains on the southwest horizon, 60 miles distant. Almost at once an arrow sign points the way along the left-branching leg of the one-way loop and, taking that fork, we see pinyon and juniper quickly supplant the grasslands. Cryptobiotic crust is well-developed along the trail, so we must stick to the trail to avoid damaging this soil-stabilizing crust.

Many trailside shrubs are identified by small signs that correspond to the trail pamphlet, including blackbrush, prickly-pear cactus, Mormon Tea, and littleleaf mountain mahogany. Each of these plants has certain site-specific environmental requirements, so they grow in different microhabitats alongside the trail.

The trail curves around the north side of a low sandstone bluff, climbing slightly and then descending onto a sandy bench to a junction at 0.25 mile (6040'). Mesa Arch lies but 30 yards away, reached via a short spur trail. The arch is unusual in that it is on the very rim of the mesa and is formed in Navajo Sandstone. Navajo rocks are usually too massive for the formation of true arches, but a vertical joint has formed in the bluff here, isolating a fin of rock in which Mesa Arch has formed.

This beautiful span frames glorious views: precipitous Buck Canyon; the great declivity carved by the Colorado River; Washer Woman Arch and its companion spire Monster Tower; bulky Airport Tower toward the southeast; and finally, the great, sky-filling summits of the La Sal Mountains on the eastern horizon.

Returning to the junction, we take the left fork of the loop, climb over a low bluff, and drop back to the trailhead after 0.5 mile. ■

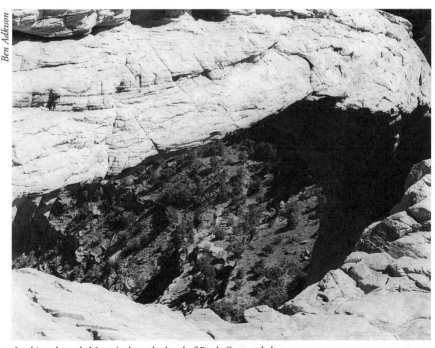

Looking through Mesa Arch at the head of Buck Canyon below

Hike 37. Murphy Point Trail

Distance	3.8 miles round trip
Elevation gain	200'
Average hiking time	2 hours
Difficulty rating	2
Child rating	2
Best seasons	April through mid-June; mid-September through October
Hazards	Steep dropoffs at the trail's end; little shade; point subject to lightning strikes

Driving to the trailhead

Follow driving directions for Hike 35 to the Island visitor center, and continue south on the park road for another 6.3 miles to a signed Y junction. Bear left (southeast) at the junction, where the sign points to Grand View Point. Just 2.5 miles from the junction a narrow dirt road branches right.

A small sign about 100 feet down that lane indicates MURPHY POINT, ROUGH ROAD. This road is very narrow, with a slightly high center, but low-slung cars can negotiate it in dry weather. It leads southwest for 0.4 mile to the confined trailhead parking area, which offers space for about three vehicles to park, but little space to turn around. Be considerate of others when you park here, and leave as much space as you can.

Introduction

This view-filled jaunt offers some of the finest views of the Green River and The Maze country obtainable from any vista point in the park. It is a pleasant jaunt, but the end of the route is obscure and sometimes uncairned as it crosses slickrock to a commanding viewpoint on the rim of Murphy Point. Nevertheless, the route is straightforward, and almost any hiker will enjoy this partly trail-less jaunt.

Description

From the trailhead (6200'), our trail heads west, following the track of a closed 4WD road. It is an easy, undulating jaunt, crossing sandy slopes studded with blackbrush, Mormon Tea, and an open woodland of pinyon and juniper.

From the end of the closed road at 1.2 miles (6160') the trail, easy to follow at first, descends slightly onto Murphy Point, a wooded slickrock promontory that juts southwest from the Grand View Point mesa.

Soon we mount Kayenta slickrock marked by widely scattered cairns, and our trail vanishes. We may encounter remnants of an old jeep road leading toward the rim. Of three points jutting out from the rim, our basic route ends at the central point on the mesa's southern rim at 1.7 miles (6080'). Hikers may wish to walk to all the points, however, for an all-encompassing vista. The westernmost point, 0.2 mile from the central point, offers perhaps the finest views of the Green River, but all of the overlooks take in a vast sweep of Canyonlands country, from the Abajo Mountains and The Needles in the southeast to the slickrock wonderland of The Maze, the Orange Cliffs, and the Henry Mountains to the southwest, and across miles of vast deserts to the San Rafael Swell on the western horizon. The broad reaches of Soda Springs Basin spread out below in the northwest, bounded by the White Rim below and the barrier of Wingate cliffs above.

Hikers who have previously seen the White Rim from viewpoints along the east edge of the mesa will notice that its cliff band is wider and thicker on the Green River side. The shallow sea along which this sandstone was deposited had its terminus near where the Colorado River is today, so the

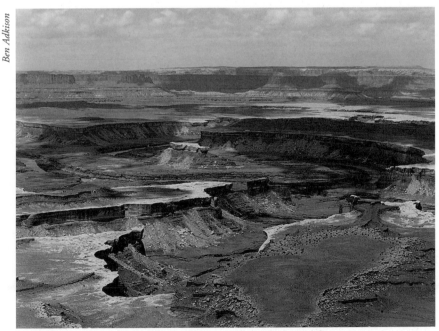

Ben Adkison

White Rim and Green River from Murphy Point. Turks Head is at left-center.

deposits had less time to accumulate there than farther west, where the sea persisted for ages.

As in all of the basins below the Island mesa, numerous mineral-exploration roads that date back to the 1950s traverse the landscape when viewed from above, although many are difficult to locate on the ground.

This viewpoint is a superb location from which to view a desert sunset. Eventually we must reluctantly pull away from the incomparable view of isolated buttes, gaping declivities, vast plateaus, and island mountain ranges, and retrace our steps to the trailhead.   ■

Hike 38. White Rim Overlook Trail

Distance	1.8 miles round trip
Elevation gain	170'
Average hiking time	1 hour
Difficulty rating	2
Child rating	1 to 2
Best seasons	April through mid-June; mid-September through October
Hazards	Steep dropoffs at the trail's end; no shade

Driving to the trailhead

Follow driving directions for Hike 35 to the Island visitor center, and continue south on the park road for another 6.3 miles to a signed Y junction, where the sign points to Grand View Point. Bear left (southeast) and after 5.1 miles from the junction, you reach a spur road branching left to a signed picnic area. Hikers turn off here and proceed midway through the picnic area for 0.1 mile to the trailhead parking area, with only four parking slots for hikers.

Introduction

The Island in the Sky is famous for far-ranging vistas, and hikers need not trek any great distance from the mesa-top roadway to enjoy them. The White Rim Overlook provides perhaps the finest view in the Island District of the 2000-foot-deep canyon of the Colorado River, and distant, awe-inspiring panoramas of Utah's rugged canyon-and-mesa country.

Description

From the trailhead/picnic area (6270'), we take the signed right-fork, a wide trail that descends just south of a broken Kayenta Sandstone rim. Drought-tolerant utah junipers form a widely scattered woodland of small, twisted trees, joined by only an occasional pinyon. Only a few wildflowers adorn the thin, sandy soil along the trail, but the yellow blossoms of haplopappus and broom snakeweed stand out among the coarse gray shrubs.

Far-ranging vistas of the canyon country accompany us all along the trail. After 0.5 mile we mount slickrock, guided by cairns. Approaching the end of the rocky promontory, we pass beneath a short but prominent pinnacle, and reach land's end at White Rim Overlook at 0.9 mile (6100'). This is the one of only two points on a trail in the Island District from which you can see the Colorado River, but only vignettes of its brush-clad banks are visible over 2000 feet below us in the river's inner gorge.

The sandy swath of the White Rim Trail 4WD road follows the edge of the broad Moenkopi bench below the mesa. The Gooseberry Campsite lies alongside that road to the north. The White Rim Sandstone forms the edge of that bench, and here in the eastern part of the park it is quite narrow and thin, pinching out entirely toward the north beneath the promontory of Dead Horse Point.

The large buildings of the Potash millsite can be viewed up-canyon, lying at the end of Utah Highway 279 southwest of Moab. Downstream, the Colorado is a wild river not crossed by another road for 80 miles south of Moab. Scattered Navajo Sandstone domes dot the surface of the Island mesa, but abruptly plunge into the basin below via the Wingate cliffs and a step-like series of softer rocks—the Chinle and Moenkopi. Save for the White Rim, the entire landscape is composed of red slopes, cliffs, canyons, and mesas. This is truly redrock country at its finest.

Our view also reaches into the depths of Monument Basin below the White Rim, where dozens of slender pillars rise from the declivity below. They are composed of the Organ Rock Shale member of the Cutler Formation, a thinly bedded and relatively soft rock. Remnants of the White Rim Sandstone cap some pillars, protecting the chimney-like rocks from rapid erosion. Much of the vista encompasses far-away landmarks such as the La Sal and Abajo mountains, and the vast array of sandstone pinnacles in The Needles to the southeast and The Maze to the southwest.

Return the way you came. ■

Hike 39. Grand View Trail

Distance	1.8 miles round trip
Elevation gain	40'
Average hiking time	1 hour
Difficulty rating	1
Child rating	1
Best seasons	April through mid-June; mid-September through October
Hazards	Steep dropoffs at the trail's end

Driving to the trailhead

Follow driving directions for Hike 35 to the Island visitor center, and continue south on the park road for another 6.3 miles to a signed Y junction where the sign points to Grand View Point. Bear left (southeast) and after 6.1 miles reach the one-way loop and parking area at the road's end.

Introduction

True to its name, the Grand View Trail offers perhaps the most all-encompassing panorama of the Canyonlands basin in the entire park. This is a good and popular trail that follows the narrow mesa among scattered trees and shrubs, ending at a prominent slickrock point that offers a commanding vista. No special skills are required to follow this justifiably popular trail, and it offers great rewards to anyone willing to park the car and walk a short distance among awe-inspiring surroundings.

Description

From the spacious parking area (6250') we should first stroll the few feet down to Grand View Overlook, where an orientation display familiarizes us with prominent landmarks seen across the vast sweep of desert that lies before us.

The signed Grand View Trail strikes southwest just short of the overlook, following the increasingly narrow promontory of Grand View Point, the southern arm of the Island in the Sky mesa. A sparse woodland of pinyons and junipers dots the slickrock of the point, their squat and gnarled forms tortured by the elements but clinging tenaciously to life. The undulating trail is embraced by broken slabs and boulders composed of Kayenta Formation rocks. Cairns lead our way where we cross slickrock. Superb vistas stretch across the vast Canyonlands basin to far-away mountains that loom like hazy mirages on the horizon.

We reach the trail's end at 0.9 mile (6240'), where large boulders are stacked upon the point, and scramble up them for an all-encompassing vista. From our vantage, we cannot see the Colorado River, but we do see the immense canyon system it has created. In the west the Green River flows placidly through Stillwater Canyon, and beyond it vast desert basins and gaping canyons rise steadily to the Orange Cliffs. Three prominent mountain ranges, the Henry, Abajo, and La Sal, as well as Boulder and Thousand Lake mountains—part of Utah's High Plateaus—rise above an endless sea of slickrock desert. Prominent Junction Butte, once part of the immense plain that existed here prior to the downcutting of the canyon network, now stands alone, filling our southward view.

We can see parts of the White Rim Trail 4WD road and a maze of uranium-exploration roads below us on either side of the point. The White Rim Sandstone forms a narrow but prominent band around the intermediate basin below the mesa. Eastward is striking Monument Basin, where a host of redrock spires, composed of the Organ Rock Shale, reach skyward from the depths of the deep canyon below the White Rim. Foregrounding the massive Abajo Mountains in the southeast are the aptly named Needles, a profusion of slickrock spires, and to the southwest is the terra incognita of The Maze. ■

Hike 40. Aztec Butte Trail

Distance	2.25 miles round trip
Elevation gain	250'
Average hiking time	1 hour
Difficulty rating	2
Child rating	2
Best seasons	April through mid-June; mid-September through October
Hazards	Short but steep slickrock scrambling near the trail's end

Driving to the trailhead

Follow driving directions for Hike 35 to the Island visitor center, and continue south on the park road for another 6.3 miles to a signed Y junction. Turn right at the junction and drive 0.7 mile to the signed Aztec Butte parking area.

Introduction

Aztec Butte is one of the more prominent Navajo Sandstone domes on the Island, and the short but scenic jaunt to its nearly flat summit reaches an all-encompassing panorama. The trail also leads past a few Ancestral Puebloan granaries, offering glimpses into a long-since-vanished culture that thrived in the region hundreds of years ago. These ancient structures crumble easily, so treat them with care and do not climb in or on them.

Description

From the trailhead (6100'), our gaze stretches across rolling grasslands, stands of pinyon and juniper, and a scattering of low-profile slickrock domes, all foregrounding the ever-present La Sal Mountains on the far northeast horizon. The trail descends gradually toward the foot of one of those domes among a variety of desert trees, wildflowers, and shrubs. Yucca soon appears in drift sand next to the trail as we reach the foot of the dome and turn north, soon skirting the eastern foot of the dome along the edge of Willow Flat's grasslands.

Shortly we curve northwest around the dome and mount a broad saddle on the edge of the grassland at 0.4 mile (6100'). At the foot of Aztec Butte, the most prominent dome in the area, we continue following cairns as we scramble up the moderately steep slickrock slopes of the dome. Erosion along the bedding planes of the Navajo Sandstone has formed small ledges that offer better footing. We quickly mount smoother slickrock and climb two steep pitches, connected by a marginal trail. Novice hikers may be intimidated by climbing steep slickrock, but good rubber-soled shoes offer a grip on the coarse sandstone.

After surmounting the summit area of the butte at 1.0 mile (6298'), we stroll northeast to the rim, where we find a low stone wall, ruins of an Ancestral Puebloan granary. Vistas from the butte are superb and far-ranging, stretching across the vast grasslands of Grays Pasture to the distant La Sal Mountains in the northeast and to the two-tiered barrier of the Book Cliffs far to the north. Closer at hand, the prominent gash of Trail Canyon lies 1000 feet below, bounded by soaring red Wingate Sandstone cliffs that are capped by scattered slickrock domes. Seasonal waters draining that canyon are destined for the Green River, a silent waterway lying in the great canyon it has carved far below in the west.

Views southeast extend as far as the forested Abajo Mountains, and lying below them are the fins and spires of the park's Needles District. South of the La Sals on the distant eastern horizon, our gaze reaches 90 miles to a few towering summits of the La Plata Mountains in Colorado. There is an abundance of cryptobiotic crust on the flat summit of the butte, so stay on the trail to avoid damaging it.

Although these vistas are magnificent, a 0.25-mile loop around the butte's rim offers still more views, as well as arches and ancient granaries. Head north past the ruin (about 3 feet high and 6 by 8 feet in dimension) and look for a faint trail just below the rim. Follow it west, quickly reaching a small, shady alcove and an arch. The ruins of another small granary lie within the alcove. The trail ahead follows a narrow ledge first west, then southwest, passing two more alcoves with ruined walls of ancient granaries. Curving around to the northwest face of the butte, we reach yet another alcove at 1.1 miles, featuring four small arches. Within the alcove are two well-preserved granaries, built of tightly fitted sandstone slabs. One of these ancient structures is cemented with red mortar, and if you look closely, finger marks in the mortar are evident. Do not climb in these structures; they are fragile and easily damaged.

Our alcove-framed view is probably much the same as the view when the Ancient Ones traveled here hundreds of years ago, as little has changed in this seemingly timeless land. Only the paved park road serves to remind us of the modern world in which we live. Perhaps they waited here for deer and bighorn sheep to hunt for food, for west of us game trails crisscross the bench below.

More fine views stretch west from our sheltered vantage point. The square-edged mesas and sheer, colorful sandstone cliffs typify the essence of the canyon country. Far to the northwest, beyond endless wooded mesas, are the uplifted flanks of the San Rafael Reef, its tilted strata rising to the highland of the San Rafael Swell. Utah's High Plateaus form the western horizon beyond the swell, rising to upwards of 11,000 feet in elevation.

To return to the trailhead, continue south along the trail from the granaries, taking great care as the narrow trail immediately skirts the abutment of a small arch, clinging to the edge of a steep dropoff. The trail then quickly regains the top of the butte and loops around the rim to rejoin the primary trail, on which we backtrack for 1.0 mile to our cars. ■

Hike 41. Whale Rock Trail

Distance	1.2 miles round trip
Elevation gain	140'
Average hiking time	30 to 40 minutes
Difficulty rating	2
Child rating	2
Best seasons	April through mid-June; mid-September through October
Hazards	Sections of scrambling over steep and exposed slickrock

Driving to the trailhead

Follow driving directions for Hike 35 to the Island visitor center, and continue south on the park road for another 6.3 miles to a signed Y junction. Turn right at the junction and drive 4.2 miles to the spacious parking area, signed for Whale Rock, on the right (north) side of the road.

Introduction

The short trip to Whale Rock offers ample rewards for a little effort: an enjoyable slickrock scramble from the mesa to the rim of Upheaval Dome, and an appreciation of the dimensions of this unusual sandstone dome. Although parts of the route along the steep slickrock slopes of the dome are exposed, handrails offer novice hikers a sense of security.

Description

From the trailhead (5710'), the gravel trail leads north, and quite soon we skirt the foot of a low slickrock hill, then begin climbing west toward the hogback crest of Whale Rock. Handrails help steady acrophobic hikers, and mortared cairns guide the way over the rock.

Upon reaching the crest, our route curves south and climbs past a display featuring an aerial view of Upheaval Dome. Soon thereafter we reach the trail's end atop Whale Rock at 0.6 mile (5850'). Looking from west to north, we realize that Whale Rock is part of the Upheaval Dome structure. Concentric rings of slickrock ridges and narrow, wooded draws nearly encircle the dome, but from our vantage point we cannot see into the dome's crater. But we can see down the cliffbound course of Upheaval Canyon, its sheer orange walls framing a memorable view of the Green River and distant mesas stretching far away toward the San Rafael Swell, some 40 miles west.

South beyond the grasslands and woodlands of the mesa, the pinnacle of Candlestick Tower stands silent guard over the redrock wilderness of Stillwater Canyon. Still farther south and southwest are the landmarks of Ekker and Elaterite buttes and the slickrock jungle of The Maze. The peaks of the Henry Mountains, 60 miles away, peek above the tilted strata of Upheaval Dome, and the ever-present La Sals dominate our view eastward over the dome-studded expanse of the Island mesa.

The gaping declivity of Trail Canyon, below us in the north, slices deeply into the mesa like a great wound in the earth. Its sheer reddish cliffs and myriad branch canyons are a delight to adventurous backpackers.

Return the way you came. ■

Hike 42. Crater View/Upheaval Dome Overlook Trails

Distance	1.8 miles round trip
Elevation gain	150 feet
Average hiking time	1 hour
Difficulty rating	2
Child rating	2
Best seasons	April through mid-June; mid-September through October
Hazards	Steep dropoffs; little shade; overlooks subject to lightning strikes

Driving to the trailhead

Follow driving directions for Hike 35 to the Island visitor center, and continue south on the park road for another 6.3 miles to a signed Y junction. Turn right at the junction and drive 5 miles to the picnic area and trailhead at the loop at the road's end.

Introduction

This short but rewarding trail is one of the most popular hikes in the Island District. It tours the south rim of unusual Upheaval Dome, offering not only dramatic views into its jumbled and eroded interior but also far-ranging vistas over canyons and mesas to lofty mountain ranges.

Description

As you begin this short hike, pick up the Crater View Trail Guide pamphlet available from the dispenser at the trailhead. It describes the rock strata you will encounter and discusses how the dome may have formed. The pamphlet, in combination with the interpretive display at Crater View, make this short trip an informative, self-guided trail.

As we leave the trailhead (5800'), we may see ravens, pinyon jays, or white-throated swifts, while a variety of lizards scurry across the trail or sun themselves on a trailside rock. After 85 yards, we pass the junction with the Syncline Loop Trail (Hike 43) and cross the slickrock of some tilted Kayenta Formation ledges. Pinyon and juniper stud the broken shelves of rock, as do shrubs typically found in this plant association, such as cliffrose, squawbush and littleleaf mountain mahogany.

As we approach the crater rim, we come to a junction at 0.2 mile (5800') where a sign indicates that one viewpoint lies 60 yards to the right via a spur trail, while another is 0.7 mile on the left-branching trail. Those who turn right will quickly mount slickrock and shortly reach the rim of the crater, where an exciting view unfolds. The floor of the crater, encircled by sheer cliffs of Wingate Sandstone, lies 1000 feet below, where the gray and red beds of the Moenkopi, Chinle, and White Rim formations are tilted and warped in a chaotic jumble of badlands hills and small peaks. Across the crater on the opposite wall, the beds of Kayenta rocks—those lying between the Navajo Sandstone domes on the rim and the sheer, reddish Wingate cliffs below—have been warped in a wave-like fashion. Interpretive displays on our slickrock viewpoint discuss various theories of the formation of the dome. Though geologists know much about the structural geology of the Colorado Plateau, the formation of Upheaval Dome continues to puzzle them.

The longer trail ahead on the left undulates over slickrock, and steps cut into the bedrock provide better footing on the steep stretches of this cairned descent. Soon we descend moderately steeply where the trail has been carved into Navajo Sandstone; before long the grade abates and we cross a pinyon- and juniper-studded flat.

We soon reach a fenced overlook at 0.9 mile (5650'), from which we enjoy an all-encompassing view of the Upheaval Dome crater. The unobstructed panorama from southwest to north takes in a vast sweep of Colorado Plateau scenery, from the Henry Mountains to Thousand Lake Mountain near Capitol Reef National Park, to the San Rafael Reef, and to the Book Cliffs. Down the cliffbound wash of Upheaval Canyon the tilted rocks of the dome in the foreground contrast dramatically with the undeformed vertical cliffs and broad platforms of Buck and Bighorn mesas, which flank the canyon. Upheaval Dome is a superb vantage point from which to enjoy a desert sunset. As shadows begin to fill the crater, the orange light of sunset paints the crater's walls in brilliant pastel shades that are unforgettable. ∎

Hike 43. Syncline Loop Trail

Distance	7.8 miles loop trip
Elevation gain	1530'
Average hiking time	4 hours
Difficulty rating	5
Child rating	3
Best seasons	April through mid-June; mid-September through October
Hazards	Trail steep and rough in places; little shade

Driving to the trailhead

Follow driving directions for Hike 35 and 42 to reach the trailhead.

Introduction

This trip is perhaps the finest half-day hike in the Island District. It descends from the rim into the backcountry, tracing a circular route around unusual Upheaval Dome, surveying landscapes ranging from pinyon-juniper woodlands to riparian areas, and from deep and rugged canyons to the cliffs bounding the Island mesa.

Description

Following the signed Crater View Trail (Hike 42) west from the road-end (5760'), we quickly encounter the Syncline Loop branching right and left. Turning left, we soon top a rise and begin a gradual descent via the syncline valley of Upheaval Dome. The valley's floor is composed of broken reddish slickrock of the Kayenta Formation, while domes of Navajo Sandstone flank us on either side. Hikers on the popular Crater View Trail are frequently seen on the skyline ridge to the north, but we'll likely see few hikers on our trail.

Fine views extend northwest, where the cliffs embracing Upheaval Canyon frame distant mesas, the far-away San Rafael Swell, and the eastern flanks of Utah's High Plateaus, their lofty environs hosting snowfields until late spring or early summer. Vegetation in this shallow valley consists of pinyon and juniper, and the shrubs commonly associated with this woodland, such as squawbush, singleleaf ash, Mormon Tea, and cliffrose.

Upon reaching the west end of the valley, we begin a switchbacking descent in the shadow of towering sandstone domes. As we continue down boulder-littered slopes, views now include the Green River. We skirt the warped strata of Upheaval Dome while enroute into the deep canyon below. The switchbacking abates, and the trail descends a steep ridge into a minor draw, which leads us to the east side of Knoll 4854. Here we switchback once again, descending a steep and sheltered chute carved into the Wingate Sandstone.

Below this chute we finally reach the canyon floor at 2.0 miles (4480') and then follow a cairned route down-canyon to our right. The increasingly deep wash has cut into layers of the Chinle Formation, which vary in color and hardness. We continue between its colorful banks, finally reaching a trail sign at 3.1 miles (4230') where Upheaval Canyon wash, draining Syncline Valley, joins from the north.

Bear right (northeast) at the junction, following Upheaval Canyon first northeast, then east to where the wash soon forks. We follow a trail climbing steep slopes with the aid of rock steps to the bench above, where we encounter a signed junction at 3.3 miles (4320'). Those who wish to explore the unique interior of Upheaval Dome, a moonscape of strangely contorted and colorful strata, can take the right fork, which leads slightly more than 1 mile, via the wash, into the eroded center of the dome.

Forking left at that junction and heading into Syncline Valley, we descend easily toward the vegetated banks of an intermittent stream, which we follow up-canyon along an undulating, boulder-strewn trail. Cottonwoods, pinyon and juniper and a variety of wildflowers, including the conspicuous blanketflower in spring, adorn the canyon bottom.

Ahead of us a cliff blocks the canyon, but a steep and rocky trail takes us around the left (west) side of that obstacle, to where we climb above the last cottonwoods and a few netleaf hackberry trees onto a sunny slope. At one point on the stiff climb, a cable offers a handhold where we cross the face of a low cliff on a built-up section of trail. The trail ahead is rather exposed, requiring some boulder hopping and the occasional use of hands.

Above this stretch, we enter the realm of steeply tilted Kayenta slickrock, above which rise domes of Navajo Sandstone. Pinyon and juniper woodlands begin to dominate the vegetation, but the damp canyon bottom hosts the greatest diversity of plants in the Island District. Cottonwoods, some quite large, thrive along the canyon's wash. Dogbane, or Indian hemp, is a white-flowered plant with fairly large, oval, green leaves. Water birch grows in tandem with false Solomon's seal and snowberry.

Our canyon eventually bends south, where it is joined by a dead-end, east-trending canyon, where alcoves and wet seeplines can be seen on its Navajo Sandstone slickrock. Presently our canyon narrows considerably between high cliffs, and cairns help guide the way. By now, pinyon and juniper have supplanted much of the lush greenery, but a few water birches persist in the narrows.

Soon we climb steeply via slickrock ledges, where numerous potholes may hold water after a good rain. The trail ahead undulates over steeply tilted ledges, dipping into and back out of the wash several times, but the hiking is easy, with only minor ups and downs. Eventually, our trail approaches the park road, then swings away from it, and we must negotiate a few more tilted ledges of the Kayenta Formation before finally joining the Crater View Trail, on which we turn left and stroll the short distance back to the trailhead at 7.8 miles.   ■

Hikes 44-50: Needles District

Hike 44. Cave Spring Trail

Distance	0.6 mile loop trip
Elevation gain	50'
Average hiking time	30 to 40 minutes
Difficulty rating	2
Child rating	2 to 3
Best seasons	April through mid-June; mid-September through November
Hazards	Steep dropoffs; two ladders that must be climbed to bypass cliffs

Driving to the trailhead

The Needles District of Canyonlands National Park lies just across the Colorado River from the Island in the Sky, but requires a roundabout drive over mesas and down deep canyons to access it. The only road into The Needles is Utah Highway 211, a paved two-lane highway branching west from U.S. Highway 191, 40 miles south of Moab and 14 miles north of Monticello. Be sure to have plenty of supplies and fuel before driving this road; Needles Outpost, 31.7 miles from U.S. 191, is your only source in the Needles area for fuel.

From the prominently signed junction of Utah 191 and Utah 211, follow Utah 211 across the mesa and down the Indian Creek valley. You reach the Needles visitor center after 32.2 miles.

Beyond the visitor center you continue straight ahead, ascending a slight grade and soon reaching a signed junction at 33 miles, where a left-branching road is signed for RANGER RESIDENCES and SALT CREEK. Turn left (southwest) here, ignoring a signed spur road to the Ranger residences after 0.25 mile. Soon we descend toward Squaw Canyon, and after 0.7 mile, turn left (east) at the signed junction with a wide dirt road. This road, which typically has a rough washboard surface, crosses brushy flats mantled in greasewood, sagebrush and rabbitbrush beneath low sandstone knolls. You pass the Split Top Group Campsite and reach the signed SALT CREEK JEEP TRAIL after 0.8 mile. Continue straight ahead, and after another 0.2 mile you reach the roadend and the Cave Spring parking area, 2.5 miles from the visitor center.

Introduction

In the Salt Creek drainage, the primary watershed of The Needles, numerous "pockets" extend away from the wash into the slickrock that surrounds it. Some of these pockets are quite large, containing isolated basins more than one square mile in extent, while others are only minor draws.

From the late 19th century until the 1970s, cattle from the Dugout Ranch grazed the grassy pockets of The Needles country. Some of the larger pockets were able to withstand intensive grazing, and they remain as grasslands today. But in the small Cave Spring pocket, cattle congregated around the precious water, and the grassland sustained irreparable damage. Now this pocket is infested with unusually large shrubs, and the Cave Spring Trail carves a swath through the shrubby pocket. Parts of the trail offer expansive vistas, and it passes a pictograph panel and well-preserved cowboy camp.

Description

A leaflet available at the trailhead describes the Cave Spring Trail, one of the four self-guided trails in the Needles District. The trail forms a loop, and arrow signs guide us along the left-hand leg of the loop as we leave the trailhead (4920').

The trail proceeds southwest through unusually tall brush, and soon curves around a slickrock promontory, entering the shade of an alcove beneath an overhanging sandstone wall. A trailside feed bin appears as we approach the fenced mouth of the alcove, wherein lies a remarkably well-pre-

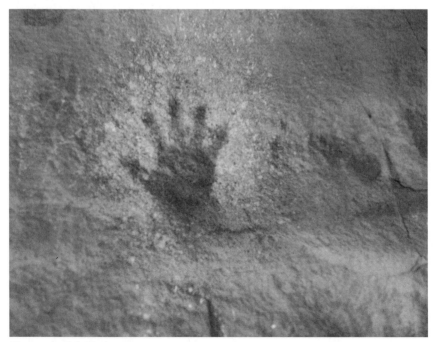

Pictographs, Salt Creek

served cowboy camp. Tables, cabinets, old cans, pots and pans, an old stove, and leather harnesses remind us of the bygone days when cowboys maintained their lonely vigil over their herds of cattle. Enjoy this historical site, but do not disturb it in any way. A seep dampens the wall behind the camp, but cowboys must have relied upon Cave Spring for water.

As we continue west beneath the overhang, we pass among squawbush and sacred datura, then stroll through an old cattle drift fence, and soon reach the deep alcove from which dripping Cave Spring issues. Its seeping waters nourish a small hanging garden of maidenhair fern and mosses. Waters collected in the porous sandstone above the vaulted ceiling of the cave issue from a seepline at the contact zone with an impermeable layer below. Over the ages, this seeping water has dissolved the cement that binds the rock together, forming a horizontal zone of weakness that eventually led to the alcove's formation.

A Fremont pictograph is near the spring, and the alcove's ceiling is blackened by the soot of countless past campfires. Not only did the Ancestral Puebloan and the Fremont people come here to drink the spring's waters, but cowboys came to establish a line camp here in this land of little moisture.

The trail continues beneath the overhang beyond the spring, then opens up in a brush-infested pocket, and shortly thereafter we reach a tall ladder, which we ascend to pass above a plunging cliff. Just ahead, after 0.2 mile, we reach a second, shorter ladder, and we ascend it out of a narrow joint and onto the gentle highland above. Curving north over the prominently cross-bedded surface of slickrock, we pass numerous soil-filled potholes hosting shrubs such as yucca, singleleaf ash, and Mormon Tea, plus pinyon and juniper. Seasonal wildflowers, including cryptantha and haplopappus, further enliven the smooth bedrock alongside the trail.

Enroute we enjoy distant views contrasting such features as the alpine peaks of the La Sal Mountains with the desert crag of North Six-shooter Peak, and broad, slickrock-embraced grassland with the cottonwood-lined wash of Salt Creek. We descend gradually, the slickrock tread giving way to soft sand as we drop into a brush-clad pocket, thickly overgrown with greasewood, four-wing saltbush, sagebrush, and rabbitbrush. Enroute we pass beneath an overhanging ledge, offering brief but welcome shade on a hot day.

Soon the pocket opens up to the east and we close the loop after 0.6 mile as we stroll down to the trailhead. ■

Hike 45. Pothole Point Trail

Distance	0.6 mile semiloop trail
Elevation gain	20'
Average hiking time	30 minutes
Difficulty rating	1
Child rating	1
Best seasons	April through mid-June; mid-September through November
Hazards	Negligible

Driving to the trailhead

Follow driving directions for Hike 44 to reach the Needles visitor center, and continue straight ahead, reaching a Y junction after 2.7 miles. Continue straight ahead at the junction, driving northwest on the Scenic Drive for 2.1 miles to the signed Pothole Point parking area on the left (west) side of the road.

Introduction

This interesting, self-guided nature trail is easy enough for novice hikers and fascinating enough to attract the seasoned hiker. Along the short, cairned slickrock trail one will find myriad potholes in the Cedar Mesa Sandstone slickrock. At certain times when conditions are ideal, the water-filled potholes are home to a variety of small, unusual creatures.

Description

Before beginning this pleasant stroll, pick up a leaflet describing potholes and the small creatures that inhabit them, available for a small donation at the trailhead (5070'). The trail initially proceeds west over corrugated slickrock among a scattering of pinyon, juniper, and various shrubs. After 150 yards the trail forks, and the two forks form a loop. To follow the loop in a clockwise direction we bear left, crossing slickrock pockmarked with innumerable potholes and passing a number of minor knolls that cap this unimposing ridge.

Most of the potholes are small and shallow, just beginning to fill with sand and clay. Hikers visiting in early spring may find them filled with water and teeming with small crustaceans, such as tadpole and fairy shrimp, snails, worms, and possibly spadefoot-toad tadpoles. All these creatures and more depend on the pothole environment, where they must complete their life cycles very quickly in the ephemeral pools.

Larger potholes with deeper soils host a few shrubs, and still larger ones host many shrubs and an occasional pinyon or juniper. All of them have a "bathtub ring" of desert varnish, formed as mineral-laden waters evaporate in the desert sun and leave behind a coating of minerals such as manganese oxide.

Potholes form from the combined action of wind and water. When water collects in a minor depression, the cementing agents that have bound the sand grains into rock there are weakened and dissolved. Once the water has evaporated, wind helps remove the loose sand, thus deepening the depression. Rainwash from downpours also helps to remove loosened sand. As this yearly cycle repeats itself, over time the pothole becomes increasingly large in depth and breadth.

Our trail eventually leads to a fine viewpoint just above the Scenic Drive, where we gaze upon a host of cliff-edged mesas, the La Sal Mountains, and the rugged Needles. Presently the trail begins to curve back toward the trailhead, passing a very short spur to a viewpoint on a trailside knob that offers a sweeping vista of Canyonlands country. Approaching the trailhead, our cairned route passes between a mushroom-shaped rock and an overhanging ledge. Both are good examples of differential erosion, where the softer, stream-deposited red beds have eroded and weathered at a faster rate than the overlying sandstone. Once we conclude the loop, we turn left and stroll back to the trailhead. ■

Hike 46. Slickrock Trail

Distance	2.4 miles semiloop plus 0.6 mile round trip to four viewpoints
Elevation gain	170'
Average hiking time	1½ hours
Difficulty rating	2
Child rating	2
Best seasons	April through mid-June; mid-September through November
Hazards	No shade; steep dropoffs

Driving to the trailhead

Follow driving directions for Hike 44 to reach the Needles visitor center, and continue straight ahead, reaching a Y junction after 2.7 miles. Continue straight ahead at the junction, driving northwest on the Scenic Drive for 3.4 miles to the signed Slickrock Trail parking area on the right (north) side of the road.

Introduction

This is a short yet delightful stroll over Cedar Mesa Sandstone slickrock, featuring panoramic vistas of canyons, cliffs, mesas, and mountains throughout its length. It's an introduction not only to plant life on the slickrock but also to the type of hiking one encounters in The Needles, where most "trails" are simply cairned routes over solid stone.

Description

Heading northeast from the trailhead (4960'), we quickly drop to a trailside box where you can pick up a leaflet (for a small donation) with a map and a brief description of the trail. Then we cross a minor wash and wind upward through the slickrock, following cairns amid pinyon and juniper. Topping a rise, we meet the first viewpoint spur trail at 0.25 mile (5050'), leading 50 feet northeast to Viewpoint #1. A grand vista stretches from Junction Butte in the northwest to the great orange cliffs that abut Hatch and Harts points and to the La Sal Mountains in the northeast. The gorge of Little Spring Canyon lies below, and to the south are the fins, domes, and spires of The Needles. Prominent North Six-shooter Peak stabs the sky toward the east, and beyond rise the wooded slopes of the Abajo Mountains.

After returning to the main trail, we continue over slickrock, following cairns to avoid walking through small, soil-filled depressions with cryptobiotic crust. Blackbrush, yucca, and Mormon Tea grow in some of the larger potholes, where ample soil has collected over the ages. At 0.5 mile (5030'), the loop trail forks, and undertaking the loop in a clockwise direction, we continue our slickrock stroll above the declivity of Big Spring Canyon on the left.

The lower walls of the canyon expose the Elephant Canyon Formation, a mostly red rock that forms ledges and low, broken cliffs. At the contact zone with the overlying Cedar Mesa Sandstone (the same rock on which we are walking) on the cliffs below we can see alkali-stained seeplines and a few small hanging gardens.

As we proceed north, we notice cross-bedding in the sandstone alongside the trail, for the light-colored bands of the Cedar Mesa were deposited as wind-blown sand. The sandstone is pockmarked with potholes (like the waterpockets of Capitol Reef) and stained with desert varnish. Littleleaf mountain mahogany is a common shrub here and on slickrock throughout the Needles District.

We reach a small trailside sign where a spur trail to Viewpoint #4 forks off to the left at 1.1 miles (5010'). This is the longest spur on the hike, 0.3 mile round trip. This route descends southwest initially, and then turns north, following ledges and winding over slickrock to the viewpoint (5000'). Big Spring Canyon's intermittently damp wash lies 600 feet below, and seeps and hanging gardens dwell on the canyon walls. Our view encompasses a vast panorama of cliffs, mesas, and canyons. Prominent among the landmarks are the fins of Ernies Country and the Orange Cliffs, Elaterite Butte and Ekker Butte in the west and northwest. Closer at hand, across the canyon of the Colorado River, are isolated Junction Butte and the vast Island in the Sky mesa. The pointed summits of the La Sal Mountains rise on the northeast skyline, while the spires of North and South Six-shooter peaks are prominent landmarks in the southeast. And of course, the banded stone fingers of The Needles form the striking slickrock landscape behind us to the south.

Once we return to the main trail, we soon reach another spur at 1.2 miles (4920') that leads only 50 yards to yet another glorious vista from Viewpoint #3, where a fine panorama of slickrock knolls, blackbrush-infested flats, cliffs, mesas, mountains, and canyons meets our gaze.

Our route ahead curves around the rim of the canyon, and at length we reach the fourth and final spur route at 1.6 miles (5000'), to Viewpoint #2. Following this spur, we descend slickrock, traverse a ledge, and then scramble to a knoll from which we have a fine view of Little Spring Canyon. There are no towering spires here, as there are in The Needles, but a host of jointed knolls instead. Again, our gaze includes the cliffs, canyons, and mesas seen before—landmarks that should presently be familiar and thus are a good means of orientation in this tangled country.

To complete the circuit, we proceed generally southwest over slickrock and across ledges while enjoying constant panoramas. Soon we close the loop 1.9 miles (5030') and bear left at the junction to retrace our steps for 0.5 mile to the trailhead. ■

Hike 47. Confluence Overlook

Distance	10.2 miles round trip
Elevation gain	1250'
Average hiking time	5 hours
Difficulty rating	5
Child rating	3
Best seasons	April through mid-June; mid-September through November
Hazards	Little shade; steep dropoffs

Driving to the trailhead

Follow driving directions for Hike 44 to reach the Needles visitor center, and continue straight ahead, reaching a Y junction after 2.7 miles. Continue straight ahead at the junction, driving northwest on the Scenic Drive for 3.5 miles to the parking area at the road's end.

Introduction

This is a memorable all-day hike leading over brushy flats, through shallow washes, and among slickrock knolls to a magnificent overlook of the joining of two great western rivers—the Colorado and the Green—and the 1000-foot-deep gorges they have carved into the Utah landscape. Although there is little elevation difference between the high and low points on the trail, the trip involves many ups and downs that add up to more than 1200 feet of elevation gain, making the trip a rigorous, all-day outing.

Description

The signed trail leads past the barricade at the roadend (4900'), and at once begins descending slickrock ledges of Cedar Mesa Sandstone into the broad, sandy wash of Big Spring Canyon. We reach the wash just upstream from a seep that nurtures lush grasses and tall, spreading cottonwoods. Once in it, cairns lead a short distance upstream to a minor branch canyon, which we begin to ascend, at times quite steeply. We climb to a slickrock notch above and west of the canyon, which frames a fine picture of distant Junction Butte. A pause here offers more good views behind us, including the broken canyon walls of Big Spring Canyon and the round shoulders of the Abajo Mountains on the far horizon.

The trail west of the notch traverses into the head of another minor canyon, where we must climb a short ladder before scaling the natural slickrock steps above. As in many areas of The Needles, the sandstone has weathered along its bedding planes, forming a stairway of minor ledges.

Above this climb we amble over the corrugated slopes of a blackbrush-clad basin, crest a minor ridge, and then traverse ledges before dipping into a small Elephant Canyon tributary. Our route follows this wash down-canyon, rimmed by low bluffs of banded sandstone.

Soon washes join our canyon from left and right, and we then leave the confines of the canyon, crossing over grassy slopes to the wide, sandy wash of Elephant Canyon. The canyon here is a striking contrast to its spire-rimmed upper reaches. Its drainage is wide and open, and a stroll up or down its course makes a rewarding diversion.

We soon leave Elephant Canyon and begin to ascend a southwest-trending branch canyon. This canyon splits into three forks near its head, and here we ascend moderately steeply via a minor ridge that divides the two left forks. Topping out on a slickrock divide, we proceed west, descending slightly at times above another small canyon. Views now reach into the heart of The Needles, where a bewildering array of colorful, slender sandstone spires forms a sawtoothed backdrop to the comparatively gentle terrain we are traversing.

The irregular outline of a redrock tower lies ahead, and we proceed toward that landmark, first descending several short but steep friction pitches, then following a sandy drainage lined with clumps of wavyleaf oak, a common denizen of sandy soils. This stint leads us past and just south of the redrock tower, beyond which we top a drainage divide.

A broad, blackbrush-infested basin now spreads before us, and we presently descend shrubby slopes on a gentle grade. Superb views stretch beyond the invisible declivity carved by the Colorado River to the hinterlands of The Maze, the Land of Standing Rocks, the Orange Cliffs, and the landmark buttes of Bagpipe, Elaterite, Ekker, and Buttes of the Cross.

At 3.2 miles (5000'), in Devils Lane, we intersect a 4WD road, which heads north and south.

Our trail crosses the 4WD road, meanders over a blackbrush-clad hill, and dips into a minor northwest-trending draw. We reach the 4WD road again at 3.9 miles (4900'), at the north end of the arrow-straight valley of Cyclone Canyon. Cyclone Canyon is a graben valley—a downdropped block of the earth's crust—and its sunken, flat bottom is thickly clad in grasses. Before the establishment of the park, visitors to valleys such as this would have encountered cattle herds from Dugout Ranch.

A sign here points to the Confluence Overlook spur road, and we stroll north on the 4WD road, quickly reaching its junction with the spur. We follow the spur west along the course of a shallow draw flanked by slickrock bluffs. After passing three south-trending draws and then winding northwest, we finally bend southwest. We ascend nearly to the head of the fourth draw, where the road ends at 4.7 miles (5030') next to a pit toilet and a CON-FLUENCE OVERLOOK sign.

The overlook is close at hand now; to get there we pass the rock barricade at the roadend, stroll past a picnic table, and follow the wash a short distance southwest up-stream, then climb west via ledges to the ridge above. Enroute, a sign warns that the overlook is unfenced, and indeed you should exercise extreme caution there. Now the trail descends gently via brushy slopes and slickrock ledges to the cluster of boulders below on the canyon rim at 5.1 miles (4900').

We can't see The Confluence until we reach the very brow of the rim. Suddenly the canyon opens up to our view, and one thousand feet below, the silty, gray-green waters of the Green River exit the confines of Stillwater Canyon and join the dark brownish waters of the Colorado River. The Green River originates 400 miles north, in Wyoming's Wind River Range, on the western flanks of the Continental Divide. The Colorado also gathers its waters from the Continental Divide, 300 miles distant in Colorado's Rocky Mountain National Park. The rivers contain the silts of the rock formations through which they have flowed, giving each river its own coloration, which varies dependent upon runoff. The grayish, sometimes reddish, waters of the Green don't immediately mix into the waters of the Colorado, but rather blend slowly for a mile or so downstream.

During low water, a broad, sandy beach adorns the riverbank. In 1869, the legendary Powell Expedition established a base camp here. Game trails follow the Green River upstream, just above the thickets of riparian woodland that hug its shores.

The mesas above the rivers are all capped by the red- and white-banded Cedar Mesa Sandstone, and we can visualize a once-continuous landscape prior to the downcutting of the rivers and their tributaries. As we gaze into the canyons below, we see the bluffs of Cedar Mesa Sandstone breaking away abruptly from the rims. Below the rims lie red and gray ledges and broken cliffs of the Elephant Canyon Formation. Near the canyon bottom is one of the oldest rock formations in all of Utah's national parks—the Honaker Trail Formation, consisting of thinly layered red cliffs and gray and reddish ledges. This band is littered with boulders fallen from above and is nearly devoid of vegetation, presenting a picture of the quintessential desert-canyon landscape. It's not unusual to see rafts floating on the gentle waters below, bound for the roaring whitewater of Cataract Canyon. From Confluence Overlook, return the way you came. ■

Hike 48. Squaw Canyon Loop Trail

Distance	7.4 miles loop trip
Elevation gain	700'
Average hiking time	3½ to 4 hours
Difficulty rating	4
Child rating	3
Best seasons	April through mid-June; mid-September through November
Hazards	Much slickrock scrambling requiring the use of both hands and feet at times; steep dropoffs

Driving to the trailhead

Follow driving directions for Hike 44 to reach the Needles visitor center, and continue straight ahead, reaching a Y junction after 2.7 miles. Turn left at the junction, and after 0.25 mile, stay left again where the right-branching road is signed for Squaw Flat Campground B and Elephant Hill. Drive through Squaw Flat Campground A for another 0.9 mile to the parking area, signed for Squaw Flat Trailhead A

Introduction

The Squaw Flat trail network offers a wide variety of highly scenic trails through the heart of The Needles. These trails can be combined into a variety of loop trips. This trip ascends the drainage of Squaw Canyon, with open grasslands and woodlands of pinyon and juniper; climbs over a slickrock divide; and returns via the wooded drainage of Big Spring Canyon.

Description

The trail leads south from the parking area in Squaw Flat Campground A (5150'), skirting a sandstone knoll and a bulletin board. After only 50 yards the trail forks left to Squaw and Lost canyons and right to Big Spring Canyon. This loop trip can be traveled in either direction, but since the following description takes the loop clockwise, we bear left.

The trail cuts a southeast-bound swath through a grassy flat studded with four-wing saltbush and a variety of seasonal wildflowers. Spires of The Needles loom ominously ahead of us, and to the northeast bulky Squaw Butte foregrounds distant views that reach as far as the great peaks of the La Sal Mountains. We enter a stand of pinyon and Utah juniper at the foot of a low sandstone slope, and quickly pass through the narrow band of trees. Mounting slickrock, we climb from cairn to cairn via the step-like bedding planes of the Cedar Mesa Sandstone. After topping out on a minor slickrock ridge, we wind among potholes while enjoying expansive vistas over The Needles and the broad Indian Creek basin—a panorama of cliffs, mesas, mountains, slickrock, and grasslands. An unusual profile of Woodenshoe Arch can also be seen atop a slickrock ridge just north of east from our viewpoint.

The trail negotiates slickrock slopes enroute to the minor wash below. We stroll through pinyon and juniper, and then climb easily to another low sandstone ridge. We now see the broad, grassy valley of Squaw Canyon, bounded by slickrock knolls, domes, buttes, and spires. An intermittent green ribbon of riparian vegetation along its wash contrasts with the drab tones of the desert vegetation that surrounds it.

Our trail undulates along the west flank of the canyon, then enters an isolated stand of spindly lanceleaf cottonwoods and reaches a signed junction with the southeast-bound trail to Lost Canyon, Peekaboo Arch, and Salt Creek, on the banks of the dry, grass-lined wash at 1.2 miles (5110').

At the junction we bear right (southwest), hiking up-canyon above the wash through a rabbitbrush-fringed grassland. Prickly pear and fishhook cactus are particularly attractive when blooming in spring, and in autumn the blooms of rabbitbrush and broom snakeweed put forth a memorable floral display. The wash banks are thick with wiregrass, which is really a rush, not a grass. Widespread throughout western North America, wiregrass is typically found in moist, saline areas along streams and in swamps and marshes.

Small cottonwoods also take advantage of subsurface moisture along the wash, and intermittent stands hug its banks, as do willows, tamarisk, and clumps of desert-olive. Wyoming paintbrush is a tall, red wildflower blooming in summer and often persisting into fall, when tansy-aster and the yellow blossoms of helianthella are in full bloom.

Beyond the wash-side stroll, the sometimes dusty trail leads into drier terrain. Soon we pass beneath an overhanging cliff, offering ample shade during the morning hours. Up-canyon, amidst riparian vegetation, a host of wildflowers enlivens the landscape, including the colorful blooms of scarlet gilia, hairy goldenaster, and evening primrose.

At a signed junction with the southeast-bound trail to Lost Canyon at 2.9 miles (5200'), we bear right, following the trail above the west bank of the wash along a sagebrush-clad bench. The head of the canyon looms before us. Bounded by tall cliffs and buttes of the red- and white-banded Cedar Mesa Sandstone and streaked with a tapestry of desert varnish, it seems an impassable barrier to further travel. Our route soon begins to ascend a side canyon to avoid that barrier. Up this canyon we see a small arch on the southwest skyline. Partway up this canyon, we cross its small wash. We scale slickrock and then traverse a pothole-covered bench beneath a soaring red, tower-capped wall.

At the southwest end of the bench, we reach a signed junction at 3.8 miles (5440') where a left-branching trail heads to Elephant Canyon. A profusion of knobs, towers, and hummocky slickrock foregrounds distant views of North Six-shooter Peak, the cliff-edged mesas of Harts and Hatch points, and the seemingly ever-present La Sal Mountains.

Bearing right at the junction, we follow cairns as we climb over steep slickrock, using friction to scale a narrow, water-carved chute. We finally mount man-made steps to the slickrock divide high above Big Spring and Squaw canyons (5520').

A well-earned pause atop this ridge reveals panoramic vistas encompassing much of the Canyonlands basin and many of its outstanding landmarks. From northwest to north we gaze beyond nearby cliffs and towers to Ekker Butte, Candlestick Tower, Junction Butte, the White Rim, and the vast cliff-edged mesa of Island in the Sky. Big Spring Canyon stretches away to the north below us, but its wash is soon lost from view amid a jumble of slickrock. At the canyon's head is a cliffbound double amphitheater. The redrock fin separating the two amphitheaters has a deep, rounded notch that is likely the remains of an ancient arch.

The Cedar Mesa Sandstone in this area is much less jointed than it is near Elephant Canyon and Chesler Park to the west. This massive sandstone forms the towers, buttes, cliffs, and knife-edge ridges that surround us. In the canyon below, the landscape is a slickrock expanse of knolls cut by shallow draws that branch from Big Spring Canyon.

From the divide, cairns lead us on a traverse of buff-toned slickrock, below which we then descend steeply, using friction on the steepest pitches between cairns. Having carefully completed the descent, we emerge onto the floor of the basin at Big Spring Canyon's head, and the trail leads us through a pinyon, juniper, and Gambel-oak woodland. The trail ahead alternates between the floor of the rocky wash and just above its east bank.

As we continue, the canyon opens up somewhat, and at 6.7 miles (5120') we meet another trail leading to Elephant Canyon, this one branching left (southwest). We bear right at the junction, climbing from the wash toward the campground. We ascend gradually along the course of a shallow draw, embraced by slickrock ridges and knobs, for 0.4 mile to the junction with the northbound trail leading to Campground B. From there we bear right, ascend a short but steep stretch of slickrock, then follow a wide ledge above the pinyon- and juniper-fringed grasslands of Squaw Flat to a cave-like gap. Pass through the gap and follow the edge of a grassy pocket to complete the circuit after 7.4 miles. ■

Hike 49. Elephant Hill to Druid Arch

Distance	10.4 miles round trip
Elevation gain	1000'
Average hiking time	5 to 5½ hours
Difficulty rating	5
Child rating	3
Best seasons	April through mid-June; mid-September through November
Hazards	Steep dropoffs; slickrock scrambling

Driving to the trailhead

Follow driving directions for Hike 44 to reach the Needles visitor center, and continue straight ahead, reaching a Y junction after 2.7 miles. Turn left at the junction, and after 0.25 mile, turn right onto the right-branching road signed for Squaw Flat Campground B and Elephant Hill. The spur to Campground B forks left after 0.25 mile, but you continue straight, soon reaching the end of the pavement. This is a good, graded, gravel road, passable to passenger cars except during or immediately following heavy rains, when runoff is likely to flow across the road. There are sharp curves, a few minor grades, and some narrow stretches that dictate careful driving.

After another 2.7 miles you reach the parking area next to picnic tables, pit toilets, and a destination and mileage sign.

Introduction

One of the largest and most intriguing arches in Canyonlands adorns the head of Elephant Canyon, in the heart of The Needles. This unforgettable hike traverses slickrock, passes through narrow joints between slickrock spires and fins, and ascends a deep, sandy wash where colorful slickrock pinnacles and domes soar hundreds of feet skyward.

Description

The signed trail wastes no time climbing south from the Elephant Hill Trailhead (5120'); we ascend through a narrow joint, then climb slabby slickrock, leveling off on the bench above. Here we stroll over sandstone and pass pockets of vegetation including pinyon, juniper, cliffrose, Mormon Tea, blackbrush, Utah serviceberry, littleleaf mountain mahogany, and wavyleaf oak. Tall, banded slickrock buttes tower above us in the west, but our view from northeast to south encompasses a dramatic panorama of the vast Indian Creek basin and the soaring sandstone spires of The Needles.

Our trail leads us ever-closer to the ranks of tall spires, and after a mile or so we reach a row of jointed fins and proceed through one of the wider joints, then descend gently through a blackbrush-clad opening. The trail ahead rises gently to a signed junction at 1.5 miles (5360') where the trail forks. An eastbound trail turns left toward the campground, and we turn right (west).

We mount slickrock, descend through a short joint, and then stroll through a small basin studded with blackbrush and scattered pinyons and junipers, with a backdrop of tall spires. Beyond the basin we descend through a longer and much narrower joint. Steep and rocky switchbacks ensue, leading us down to the sandy wash of Elephant Canyon and another signed junction at 2.1 miles (5200').

Hikers bound for Chesler Park (Hike 50) will continue straight ahead, climbing the sandy wash bank to the west, but we turn left (south) and begin hiking up the sandy, rocky wash of Elephant Canyon. The trail ahead alternates between the wash and its banks. Tall, red- and white-banded fingers of stone rise above the canyon's bulging slickrock walls.

At 2.9 miles (5272'), we come to a junction where a prominent canyon branches southeast. A trail heads left here to Big Spring Canyon. We bear right at the junction, continuing up Elephant Canyon. The ensuing stretch is much the same as the last, following either the rocky wash or its wooded banks upstream.

We reach another junction at a southwest-trending canyon at 3.4 miles (5300'), where we continue straight ahead. Our route follows the wash south, mostly over slickrock, as we proceed farther into the increasingly narrow canyon.

After another 1.25 miles, where we reach a sign indicating Druid Arch, we leave the confines of the wash and begin scrambling over slickrock. We ascend a minor gully, shortly reaching a narrow ledge about 100 feet above the gorge. Our route follows the ledge up-canyon to a short steel ladder and a handrail that allow safe passage over the bulging slickrock. Above that obstacle we climb a steep gully, finally leveling off very near the head of Elephant Canyon.

The cairned route apparently ends here at 5.2 miles (5800') beneath towering Druid Arch. Some hikers proceed a bit farther for a close-up view, although the route is hazardous. The arch bears a resemblance to a huge, long-legged pachyderm, but its name was probably derived from its likeness to stone monuments at Britain's Stonehenge. ("Druid" refers to an ancient Celtic religious order.)

The arch is formed in a narrow fin projecting into the amphitheater at the canyon's head. Its two openings are tall, narrow, nearly vertical slits, probably formed along vertical joints, many of which lace the rocks of the fin, splitting the rock into a number of large slabs. A thin, red, shaley bed lies beneath the openings, but this stratum does not appear to have played a role in the development of the spans. The fin is composed of a hard, buff-toned sandstone layer of the Cedar Mesa, and has a dark-brown patina of desert varnish. Both openings are also coated with desert varnish, and this coat of minerals takes a long time to develop. The top of the larger span, formed above a horizontal joint in the fin, is angular and does not bear a coat of varnish, indicating the relatively recent enlargement of the arch.

The headwaters amphitheater of Elephant Canyon is pure slickrock. Tall cliffs—some sheer, others bulging—rise to a skyline of domes, towers, and pinnacles, some a full 600 feet above the canyon floor. Gazing down-canyon, our view stretches beyond ranks of tall spires to the distant mesa of Island in the Sky and the prominent monolith of Candlestick Tower. From Druid Arch, retrace your steps to the trailhead.   ■

Hike 50. Elephant Hill to Chesler Park

Distance	6.0 miles round trip
Elevation gain	920'
Average hiking time	3 hours
Difficulty rating	3
Child rating	2 to 3
Best seasons	April through mid-June; mid-September through November
Hazards	Slickrock scrambling; little shade

Driving to the trailhead

Follow driving directions for Hike 49.

Introduction

The spire-rimmed, nearly circular grasslands of Chesler Park encompass more than 600 acres of gentle, open terrain—a delightful change in a region dominated by seemingly endless expanses of slickrock and deep, yawning canyons.

This trip follows the most direct route to Chesler Park, and it can be taken as a round trip, or extended by following a circuit around the park, or by looping back into Elephant Canyon via the trail along the eastern edge of the park.

Description

From the Elephant Hill Trailhead (5120'), we follow the first 2.1 miles of Hike 49 to the first trail junction in Elephant Canyon. Following the sign pointing to Chesler Park, we climb west up the sandy bank of Elephant Canyon's wash, then dip into a minor wash and ascend its opposite bank.

Our route climbs broken ledges while heading into a shallow draw. Soon the trail zigzags upward over ledges and among boulders, emerging onto a bench backdropped by towering spires. Chesler Park lies beyond the spires in the southwest, but to get there our trail must first find a passable route between them. We skirt their base as we stroll easily across the bench, enjoying fine views of a profusion of slender stone fingers thrusting skyward.

Reaching a signed junction at 2.8 miles (5540'), we turn left and ascend a boulder-filled gully formed in a joint between two soaring spires. The 100-foot climb is short but steep; from the top (5640') our gaze stretches north over miles of slickrock. The trail then descends gradually among low sand hills, and soon the broad, grassy expanse of Chesler Park spreads out before us.

Upon reaching a junction at 3.0 miles (5550'), we ponder our options. We can end the hike here, perhaps finding a nearby slickrock knob upon which to enjoy the panorama across this spreading grassland, or we can consider following longer trails, extending the hike into an all-day outing.

Option 1: The trail that turns left (southeast) climbs a sandy rise, then skirts the east edge of the park. A fine viewpoint rests on the rim high above slickrock-bound Elephant Canyon. From the viewpoint, the trail turns southwest and descends gradually to a junction just east of the nest of spires that rises like an island in the middle of Chesler Park. At this junction, 1.3 miles from the previous one, turn left to follow the 1.1-mile trail into Elephant Canyon.

The trail proceeds northeast, passes through a fin-rimmed gap, and levels off on a flat below. Presently, the trail dips into the head of a draw, which you briefly follow southward downhill. Soon you leave the draw to wind northeast along a narrow slickrock ledge while searching for a way into Elephant Canyon below. The traverse ends amid potholed slickrock, and you now descend into another draw, sometimes using friction to descend on steep sandstone. But soon it becomes too steep, and you then traverse first east, then south, descending via discontinuous ledges and finally reaching the trail in Elephant Canyon (5300') after 30 minutes or so of rugged hiking from the previous junction.

To complete the circuit, follow Elephant Canyon to the left (north), heading down the wash for 1.3 miles to a junction, then turning right (northeast) and backtracking for 2.1 miles to the trailhead.

Option 2: To circumnavigate this sea of desert grass, bear right at the junction, following the trail between the grassy park and a row of tall spires soaring 400 feet above in the north. The trail proceeds into rocky terrain and leaves the grassland behind. Fine views reach across the spread to wooded mesas in The Grabens area of the Needles District and to the Orange Cliffs and Henry Mountains on the far horizon.

The trail winds into and out of several draws, passes over blackbrush-clad slopes, and before long reaches a short, narrow joint. Beyond the joint our route undulates over slickrock and soon reaches another signed junction, at 3.9 miles (5450'). There you bear left (south-southwest) toward the 4WD road in the graben valley below. That valley is flanked by ranks of pinnacles, and above it to the west is the grassy, brushy expanse of Butler Flat. Beyond are more spires and the broad slopes and high, wooded mesas in the far southwest reaches of the Needles District.

The trail descends into a rocky draw, then levels in an open flat. Soon you intercept a 4WD road at 4.5 miles (5260') along the banks of Chesler Canyon's wash. Follow the sandy road southbound, as it crosses the wash

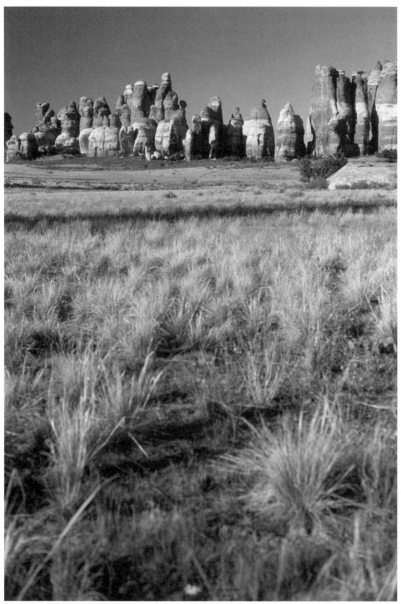

Spires of slickrock embrace the grasslands of Chesler Park

and climbs a hill. It descends to a junction at 4.7 miles (5280'), becoming rough and rocky on the way.

At the junction you turn left, where a sign indicates CHESLER PARK TRAILHEAD. Skirt grass- and brush-clad hills and sandstone knolls while following Chesler Canyon southeast upstream. Here exotic cheatgrass dominates among remnant bunches of native grasses, the result of decades of grazing on fragile grasslands by the Indian Creek Cattle Company.

At the roadend at 5.2 miles (5350'), you encounter pit toilets, a picnic table, and the beginning of the Joint Trail, one of the most exciting routes in the Needles District. The trail at once climbs a hill east of the roadend, drops into and crosses a sandy wash, and then climbs steadily toward the jumble of slickrock that lies ahead. Soon you enter a cavernous tunnel eroded into an east-trending joint. Beyond this rockbound hallway you turn abruptly north, following an increasingly narrow joint that is barely 2 feet wide in places. Some hikers may feel claustrophobic within the confines of the joint.

Eventually you exit the joint and climb a rock stairway to a signed junction at 5.8 miles (5550'). For a grand view of Chesler Park, take the right fork, signed for a viewpoint. Along this 0.1 mile diversion, you follow a brushy draw and scale slickrock, with the aid of steps cut into the smooth rock, to a commanding viewpoint atop a slickrock knoll (5600'). From north to east, the pinnacle-rimmed grasslands of Chesler Park spread out before you. Westward lie the Orange Cliffs, the splintered crown of Elaterite Butte, and the slickrock wilderness of The Maze. The Doll House is the prominent cluster of pinnacles rising above the southeast corner of The Maze.

Returning from that diversion, follow the eastbound trail as it skirts the south margin of Chesler Park. This trail rises gradually, winding along the foot of the soaring pinnacles to the south. Soon the trail curves northeast toward the cluster of spires that punctuate the spreading grassland, and you meet a northwest-bound trail leading to three designated campsites. There is a historic cowboy line camp midway along the foot of this slickrock island, including some old inscriptions on the rock behind it. Opposite that spur trail is another, shorter path leading to yet another campsite east of the trail.

Strolling past the spur trails, you soon reach a junction at 6.6 miles (5620') with the trail mentioned in Option 1, along the east edge of Chesler Park. You bear right (east) toward Elephant Canyon. Refer to the last two paragraphs of Option 1 for a description of your return route. ∎

Hikes at a Glance

Hike Number and Name	Distance (miles)	Difficulty rating	Child rating
Zion National Park			
1 Watchman Trail	2.9	3	2
2 Emerald Pools Trail	2.1	2	2
3 West Rim Trail, Grotto Picnic Area to Scout Lookout and Angels Landing	3.8–4.8	4–5	3
4 Weeping Rock to Hidden Canyon	2.2	3	3
5 Riverside Walk, Orderville Canyon	2.0–6.4	1–4	1–3
6 Canyon Overlook Trail	1.0	2	2
7 Pine Valley to Northgate Peaks Overlook	5.0	3	2–3
8 M. Fork Taylor Creek to Double Arch Alcove	5.6	3	3
Bryce Canyon National Park			
9 Queens Garden Trail	3.4	3	2
10 Navajo Loop Trail	1.5	3	2
11 Peekaboo Loop Trail	5.0	4	3
12 Bristlecone Loop Trail	1.0	2	1–2
13 Water Canyon, Mossy Cave	1.0	1	1–2
Capitol Reef National Park			
14 Chimney Rock Loop Trail	3.5	3	2–3
15 Fremont Gorge Viewpoint Trail	4.4	4	3
16 Fremont River Trail	2.5	2	1–2
17 Grand Wash	4.4	2	2
18 Old Wagon Trail	4.0	4	3
19 Capitol Gorge Trailhead to The Tanks	1.8	2	1
20 Golden Throne Trail	4.0	4	3
21 Hickman Bridge	1.9	2	2
22 Rim Overlook/Navajo Knobs Trail	9.0	5	3
23 Surprise Canyon	2.0	3	3
24 Headquarters Canyon	3.0	3	3
25 Halls Creek Overlook to Brimhall Bridge	4.6	5	3
Arches National Park			
26 Park Avenue	0.9	2	2
27 Balanced Rock Trail	0.3	1	1
28 North Window, Turret Arch, and South Windows Trail	up to 1.1	1	1–2
29 Double Arch Trail	0.4	1	1

Hike Number and Name	Distance (miles)	Difficulty rating	Child rating
30 Delicate Arch Trail	3.0	3	3
31 Delicate Arch Viewpoint	1.4	2	2
32 Sand Dune and Broken Arches	1.6-1.8	2	1-2
33 Devils Garden Trails	1.6-7.2	1-3	1-3
34 Tower Arch Trail	3.4	3	2-3

Canyonlands National Park–Island District

35 Neck Spring Loop Trail	5.3	3	3
36 Mesa Arch Loop Trail	0.5	1	1
37 Murphy Point Trail	3.8	2	2
38 White Rim Overlook Trail	1.8	2	1-2
39 Grand View Trail	1.8	1	1
40 Aztec Butte Trail	2.25	2	2
41 Whale Rock Trail	1.2	2	2
42 Crater View/Upheaval Dome Overlook Trails	1.8	2	2
43 Syncline Loop Trail	7.8	5	3

Canyonlands National Park–Needles District

44 Cave Spring Trail	0.6	2	2-3
45 Pothole Point Trail	0.6	1	1
46 Slickrock Trail	2.4-3.0	2	2
47 Confluence Overlook	10.2	5	3
48 Squaw Canyon Loop Trail	7.4	4	3
49 Elephant Hill to Druid Arch	10.4	5	3
50 Elephant Hill to Chesler Park	6.0	3	2-3

Difficulty rating: 1–easiest; 5–hardest.
Child rating: 1–suitable for toddlers; 2–suitable for children 6–8 years; 3–suitable only for well-conditioned kids older than 9–10 years.

Index

Utah's National Parks

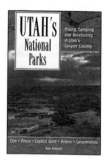

124 hikes in Utah's most spectacular parks

RON ADKISON

$17.95, 2nd edition, 2001
432 pages, 6 x 9
ISBN 0-89997-242-X
UPC 7-19609-97242-6

This book covers Zion, Bryce, Capitol Reef, Arches, and Canyonlands. Discover soaring sandstone cliffs, ancient rock-art, sun-baked desert, and open woodlands of pinyon and juniper. Up-to-date trail descriptions and campground information are featured in this new edition of *Utah's National Parks*. The trips range from brief strolls to demanding, cross-country backpack treks illustrated with photos and drawings. Also the author gives information on desert geology, plants and animals, and a topographic map for each hike.

Rock-Art of the Southwest

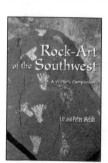

A Visitor's Companion

LIZ AND PETER WELSH

$14.95, 1st edition, 2000
176 pages, 5 1/2 x 8 1/2
ISBN 0-89997-258-6
UPC 7-19609-97258-7

The who, what, where, when, and how of rock-art. This richly illustrated book will guide you to 28 outstanding rock-art sites in 7 states, and teach you about art styles and the cultural groups that created them. Includes a resource guide to continue your exploration.

Utah Byways

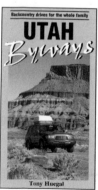

60 Trips Including Canyonlands, Arches, and Capitol Reef National Parks

TONY HUEGEL

$16.95, 2nd edition, 2000
208 pages, 5 x 9
ISBN 0-89997-263-2
UPC 7-19609-97263-1

·Drive the pathway of the historic transcontinental railroad or cover the routes of the Pony Express and Overland Stage. Gaze at rock art in Canyonlands and ascend majestic mesas. This book will be your guide.

Contact Wilderness Press to order these related titles
(800) 443-7227   mail@wildernesspress.com
www.wildernesspress.com

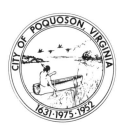

POQUOSON PUBLIC LIBRARY
POQUOSON, VIRGINIA